3rd Opinion on Prostate Cancer

A Guide to Knowing Your Options

Jessie Wright

Tate Publishing & *Enterprises*

Published by Tate Publishing & Enterprises, LLC
127 E. Trade Center Terrace | Mustang, Oklahoma 73064 USA
1.888.361.9473 | www.tatepublishing.com

Tate Publishing is committed to excellence in the publishing industry. The company reflects the philosophy established by the founders, based on Psalm 68:11,
"The Lord gave the word and great was the company of those who published it."

Cover design by Tyler Evans
Interior design by Blake Brasor

Published in the United States of America

ISBN: 978-1-61566-021-6
Medical, Oncology
10.06.14

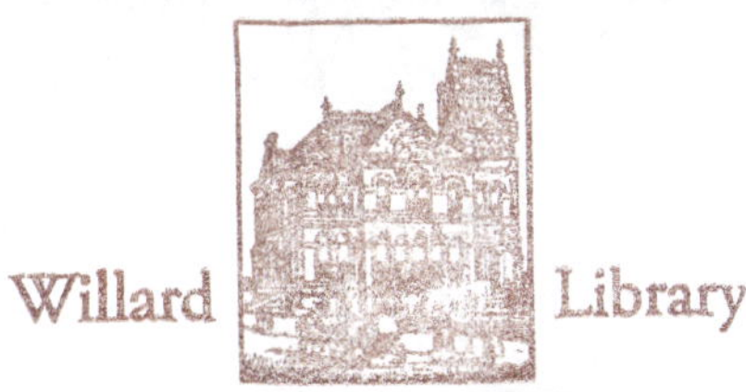

Table of Contents

Disclaimer

Although the information in this publication has been verified through reliable sources, both the author and publisher assume no responsibility for any errors, omissions or misunderstanding of the materials in this book. The author is not in the medical field nor can make any diagnosis of your state of prostate.

This book is based on author research and experiences. It has not been read or evaluated by a medical profession and should not be relied upon for medical advice replacing your physician's diagnosis.

Before accepting any treatments suggested in this book, consult with your internal Doctor and use your own judgment.

Your judgment and decision is ultimately what dictates the course of action and you agree to hold both the author and Tate Publishing's harmless from any claims valid or not.

Introduction

This book is written to empower and encourage you to take the next step in searching for the real truth as to whether you really have prostate cancer or not, despite the fact that you have received two sets of opinions from two different doctors, and two pathologists, confirming that you, indeed, do have prostate cancer. This book provides the information you need to understand what the doctors and specialists are telling you as you seek a concrete diagnoses.

As you read this book, you will find that the medical professionals can and will make a variety of undisclosed mistakes. What happened to me after being diagnosed with a prostate cancer with the Gleason score of 8 (with 10 being the worst case) will prepare you for what lies ahead?

The negligent failure to correctly diagnose prostate cancer by urologists, who rely on pathology reports, is an appalling error that must stop. Hospitals and urologists must take responsibilities for their negligence and disclose their mistakes that may cause a lifetime suffering to their patients. When these sorts of mistakes are made, it is not the patient's fault in selecting an inadequate urologist, but it is certainly the urologist's fault in selecting inadequate pathologists and laboratories that produce faulty interpretations of the biopsy results in the first place.

I certainly hope that this book will inspire the American Medical Association to require urologists to pass the same tests required of pathologists to be able to interpret the biopsy results. In order to provide an accurate diagnosis, an urologist not only needs to consider the symptoms reported by patient, but be able to review and analyze the patient's biopsy report. Just knowing the symptoms is not sufficient in order to render an appropriate diagnosis. One must include all of the information available which includes, but is not limited to, reading biopsy reports.

Humans, just like cars, can be recalled. You may laugh, but it is true. If you had surgery to remove your prostate, just to find out several months later that you did not have cancer, how would you feel? If you were recalled, just like thousands of other patients, because an unnecessary surgery was conducted, you would definitely be a part of a class lawsuit action against this kind of practice. There is no difference between this and amputating your right leg instead of your left leg by mistake.

A variety of aspects in misdiagnosing prostate cancer will be under the microscope in this book. You will be given the facts to assess your realistic options including minimally invasive surgery and gene therapy. The knowledge that you will receive, combined with your faith and common sense, will determine your ultimate option and final outcome.

Throughout this book I will reiterate on purpose a few highly important points as they are crucial for some readers to retain.

Currently urologists rely on the pathologists to read the biopsy slides and often are unable or unwilling to double check the readings they've received from the pathologists after they receive their report from the laboratory of their choice. Gruesome consequences of such process is that if a pathologist in that laboratory makes a mistake interpreting your biopsy slides, you will be sent to an unnecessary surgery; a surgery that will produce income for both the surgeon and the hospital, and be potentially fatal for you.

If you trust your physician one hundred percent and are unwilling to obtain a second, let alone a third opinion, in a diagnosis of your prostate cancer, this book is not for you.

How well do you know yourself when it comes to catastrophic news? What would you do if your urologist told you, that you have prostate cancer? Would you downright trust his judgment?

Just because an opinion comes from a professional, it doesn't mean that the opinion is accurate and trustworthy. There will always be a risk when putting your health into another person's hands, but that risk can be minimized by your common sense, experience and willingness to learn about your new condition without blindly trusting what you were told by a medical professional. Professionals are here to give you their opinion, but the ultimate decision is yours not theirs. Would you let your attorney or your accountant make your business decisions? Would you let your medical professional make a life threatening (or saving) decision for you? It is something to contemplate.

To be successful in business and personal life it is helpful to have a set of principals and stick to them in any circumstances. For example, let's take a principle of not accepting a first offer or bid. This is most important when reviewing medical advice from all sources. Would you agree? When remodeling a house or repairing your car, do you accept the first bid? Or do you seek competitive bids? How many bids will you seek prior to a final decision? One ... Two ... Three?

By the same token, would you not do the same when it comes to opinions from medical doctors and pathologists? This is your life, how much is it worth to you? These are questions necessary for considering medical treatment. Is your life's value equal to a car's, or a home's? Ultimately, it is your decision, and your decision would be best served based upon all available information.

Prostate cancer is a serious matter, especially when your doctor shocks you with a diagnosis of rapidly growing prostate cancer. While reading this book you can kick back, laugh and lean at the same time, while keeping in mind that this is a very serious subject and your knowledge can change the outcome in your life.

This book is intended to trigger your questioning, researching and learning which should lead you to the right path. Since most of the research is included here, all you need to do is to follow through.

Like all humans, professionals can make mistakes, but it becomes appalling when you learn that many unnecessary surgeries conducted by medical professionals have been instigated by an ulterior motive, just like a greedy repair man would suggest an unnecessary job to make extra money.

You may select the best surgeon the money can buy, but if you do not have the correct diagnosis, which includes an accurate pathology report, you may end up with impotence and a leaky faucet after the surgery. We will discuss all types of treatments that are available in both the United States and abroad.

Chapter

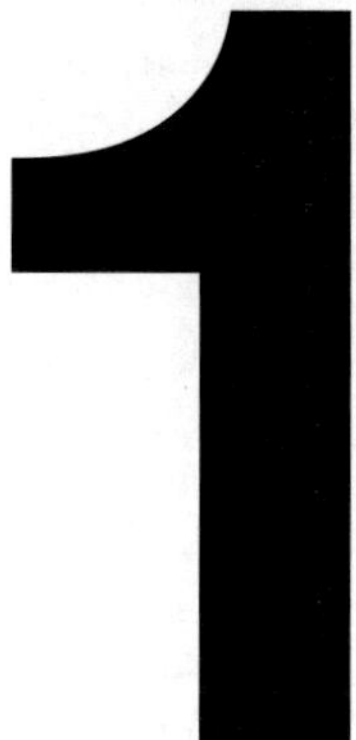

What Do You Know About Your Prostate? Where Does It All Begin? Signs and Symptoms of BPH

Do you know where your prostate gland is, and what it is for? According to Random House, it is of Greek origin and translates as: "what stands before" Your prostate lies just below the bladder surrounding the top part of the urethra, which is the tube that drains your precious urine from your precious bank, the bladder.

This book will reveal, with a twist of fun, my research not just for prostate cancer but also for bladder and bone cancer, as they are very much related. This book is also designed to give you enough information to facilitate information needed in order to clearly communicate with your physician.

The size of your prostate is the size of the pea when you are born, and it grows to be the size of a walnut. I don't know about you, but for me, things that are a high priority must be visible right in front of me at all times in order to maintain my attention. If you or someone you care about has been diagnosed with prostate cancer, the next time you are in a grocery store, buy a few walnuts. Place one in your pocket, one next to your bed, one on your desk, one in the bathroom, and one on your office desk. If someone asks you why you are keeping them there, you can tell them that in such a short time you must learn so much in order for you to resolve the issue, and the walnut is a constant reminder of this. The walnut is simply a reminder to pay attention to your prostate health.

Your prostate gland, through glandular tissue, produces the seminal fluid that transports and nourishes your sperm without which your wife cannot get pregnant. Shooting blank is another way to describe it, if that function of prostate is out of order. The second known thing that your prostate does is that by using its secretions, it keeps the lining of urethra moist. Without this function, your urine will either have difficulties transferring to the bladder, or it will remain in the prostate gland for some time, and we don't want that, do we?

What is BPH? It is one of the common prostate disorders known as benign prostatic hyperplasia (BPH), or benign prostate enlargement. It is a noncancerous condition of an unknown cause. This slow growth of the prostate occurs in approximately 70 to 80 percent of men. It is the only organ that continues to grow slowly after the age of twenty-five. Now, if we could just shrink that little rascal with whatever ways you can imagine, you would not have BPH.

In BPH, the prostate gland can increase in size from twenty grams (0.71 ounces), which is the average size of the prostate in younger men, to as large as 150 grams (5.31 ounces), and that is almost eight times of the normal size. The size of my prostate at the age fifty-three was forty-nine grams. As the prostate grows, it constricts the urethra, possibly causing a partial obstruction and invasion of the bladder. Such obstruction may lead to bladder wall thickening. In other words, my bladder tells my prostate, "Hey, buddy, stop pushing or I will block the river." That's when the urination problems begin.

Once your river, at the command of your bladder, gets partially blocked, it can bring certain surprises and symptoms such as frequent urination, constant or semi-constant nighttime urination, a feeling of urgency to urinate, difficulty emptying the bladder, and a weak urinary river stream.

You will learn certain steps that you can take to stop the growth of your walnut, recognize errors and mistakes made by urologists, misreading and misdiagnoses of the prostate biopsy, the available treatments such as herbs, medicines, minimally invasive and full-blown surgeries that are available in the United States and around the world. This information will help you make an intelligent decision when it comes to being so close to that surgery knife.

Once diagnosed with prostate cancer, what most patients typically do is rush to make a choice of a type of surgery to undergo and they become so short-sighted that they don't think "Hey, wait a minute, what if they made a mistake? What if the enlargement is not cancerous?" One of my principles in life is "I will cross the bridge when I come to it". Reading this book in its entirety will help you cross that bridge.

Once you know that your prostate is enlarged and you have been given the confirmation from the digital rectal exam, DRE, or what I call 'the enjoyable finger test," when the doctor inserts a gloved finger in your behind with a smile, it is time to be concerned. The next step, depending on your urologist's recommendation, is a biopsy and prescription for medications that will be able to shrink the size of that little rascal. Medications should smooth the muscles in the prostate gland alleviating the bladder obstruction of the river.

As much as you may not like to hear this, the finger test in my opinion must be repeated at least three times by three different doctors just to know if their fast fingers can detect the same nodules or bumps. Since this book is about a principal of getting a third opinion, you will see how important it is to have at least three sets of opinions without disclosing the results to others to ensure untainted second and third opinions.

Why?, you may ask. What if you take the finger test with the first doctor and he finds out that you have a BPH and a nodule? Telling the other two doctors this information may compromise the results of their exams since their opinion will be influenced by the results you have disclosed to them. I took the finger test four times! And no, it was not enjoyable. Finger test number one showed that I had BPH but no nodule. Finger test number two in Europe confirmed it. Finger test number three by Dr. Leonard Marks showed that I had BPH and a nodule of two millimeters. Finger test number four confirmed the BPH but not the nodule. Having a nodule did not worry me since it does not necessarily equate to having cancer. What is the next step?

First, let's get technical and go deeper into the subject. Let us talk about prostate gland related disorders. Prostate cancer (prostatitis) is an inflammatory condition of the prostate that is most common in men ages twenty to fifty.

There are two broad classes of prostatitis: nonbacterial and bacterial. Nonbacterial prostatitis is the most common form of prostatic inflammation. It causes pelvic pain, which we will discuss later, problems with urination, discomfort after ejaculation, and lower back pain. These are the symptoms to watch and remember. Since I did have excruciating back pain, I got alarmed that it was related to nonbacterial prostatitis or bone cancer, but luckily, this was a false alarm since it was simply my lower back arthritis acting up. Having been told that I had a Gleason 8 prostate cancer which may spread into my pelvis, and required and a bone scan, was not fun.

In bacterial prostatitis, which may be sexually transmitted, a bacterial infection in the prostate gland leads to swelling, pain, and difficulty in urinating. The penis may release bacterial fluid, and blood may appear in the urine. In some cases, bacterial prostatitis can cause a severe infection throughout the body, producing a dangerously high fever. Bacterial prostatitis is treated with antibiotics, but sometimes all of the infection cannot be eliminated from the prostate gland, and some men develop a chronically infected prostate. Obviously, to men that are faithful to their wives and men that believe in sex only after marriage, this or AIDS is not a condition to worry about and we won't worry about it in this book either.

In nonbacterial prostatitis a cause of which, as of the date of the publishing of this book, remains unclear, symptoms often remind those of bacterial prostatitis and include pain in lower back and genital area, painful urination and ejaculation, frequent urge to urinate and blood in urine. Recent evidence suggests that nonbacterial prostatitis may be caused by bacteria that are present in the middle of a prostate but cannot be detected by conventional diagnostic techniques.

There is no known cure for nonbacterial prostatitis and patients are treated with medications ranging from antibiotics to antispasmodics. The success of such treatments varies widely, and in many cases, men must live with the symptoms of prostatitis.

Signs and Symptoms of BPH

The prostate gland is the only organ that continues to grow in men after the age of twenty-five. Over 90 percent of all prostate cancers are from the outer part of the prostate gland, which, as discussed earlier, can be detected by 'the enjoyable finger test,' (DRE). And although the doctor's finger may not necessarily be your favorite size, it is still lubricated passing through your rectum, and the doctor can feel for bumps, nodules, or abnormalities. Almost everyone that I interviewed for this book told me that it was an embarrassing experience and there is nothing sexual about it. This test is not really an accurate measurement with certainties, but it does save lives.

Within a period of a year, I had four finger tests with four different doctors, one in Europe and three in California. Only one doctor, Dr. Leonard Marks in UCLA Medical Center, was able to notice a nodule that was unusual.

Why four finger tests, you ask? No, I am not gay, and no, I did not enjoy it. You see, doctors make mistakes, especially when they are detecting a bump the size of two millimeters, which was the size of my nodule. The smaller the size, the harder it is to be detected.

Signs and symptoms of BPH include difficulty starting urination and weak urine stream, which is very noticeable. It feels like some kind of blockage. Another symptom is stopping and starting and or dribbling at the end of urination. I had these symptoms, but when it came to the main symptom of BPH, a frequent need to urinate with increased frequency at night, I had no urge to do so. Having not been able to empty my bladder always bothered me, and having excess urine in the bladder is dangerous for possible infection caused from bacteria. Urinary tract infections and blood in the urine are the two final symptoms that I did not have. Do you have them?

At what point do you need medical advice and care?

You ask for legal advice from attorneys only when you have a legal situation. Likewise, you should seek medical advice when the symptoms are troublesome and pose a health threat. Your symptoms could be early warnings of a more serious condition such as prostate cancer, bone cancer, lung cancer, heart issues, diabetes, kidney stones or bladder infection.

In my opinion, legal or medical advice is just that - advice. I realize, doctors attend medical schools, and not all of them are carless or sloppy. Nevertheless, their advice remains simply advice more, not nothing. You must remain the ultimate decision maker based upon the advice provided by three separate medical professionals.

Let me give you a couple of examples. When you pay the retainer fee for your attorney and he finally gives you his opinion of the case, don't you ask the obvious question? "What do you think I should do?"

When the physician finally sits down with you and tells you what has been detected, it is important not to confuse yourself with what the physician diagnosed, but to know if the diagnosis is correct. When you ask the same question: "What do you think I should do?" What do you think their response is going to be? They will not tell you, "Oh, yes, check into the hospital for urgent surgery," unless it is a life-and-death situation. Their response will be to get a second opinion. They will even refer you to other doctors; the only problem is that they will refer you to a doctor with the same mind frame as theirs and if they share the same biopsy results, their diagnosis will be the same. The surgeon that my fourth doctor referred me to confirmed that my Gleason score was an eight, and suggested for me to go into surgery as soon as possible. The same night it dawned on me that he had reviewed the same pathology report used in prior diagnoses. His confirmation was not based upon new report, so of course he would confirm my Gleason score. If that he had said, "Let's get these slides looked at by another pathologist or let's take another biopsy," I would have felt confident in proceeding with that surgeon.

If that's the case, what do you do?

Learn and digest this book as quickly as possible to increase your knowledge. This will provide you with a powerful tool should you ever find yourself in this position.

Let's talk about the three types of candidates for prostate cancer. Are you married? You are more likely to experience BPH than singles. There is no evidence that supports the common denominator between married and single men attributing to BPH. This is unknown to us as of the date of publishing this book. My argument for married men having more risk of having BPH surely may not be due to sexual activities, as the percentage of married men versus single men, when it comes to statistics of sexual activities, is unknown. You are right, less sex, less chance of BPH, but no, do not stop having sex just yet as those findings are still primitive.

If you are an African American male, your risk of having a BPH is at least 50 percent higher than Caucasian men.

Are you an Asian man? You are lucky! BPH is more common in American and European men than Asian men.

If you have a family history of prostate cancer, pay attention! This book will tell you why you should be under more monitoring than any other candidates.

Below are the six minor lifestyle changes that will at least help to control the symptoms of BPH and keep your condition in the status quo.

1. If you have frequent urination and must get up several times at night, then you must stop drinking between the hours of six and eight at night, depending on, of course, the time you go to bed. I did not have this issue due to a larger capacity of my bladder, which was 49 cc. You may not have this symptom either and since it boils down to a bladder capacity, you must check the size of the bladder and compare it with a normal size of bladder for your age, weight, and height.
2. Try not to keep a full bladder for a long time and go to bathroom at the last minute. I had this tendency as in between meetings and

traffic I kept holding it in, especially during long trips.

3. Coffee and alcohol will increase urine production. If you can't cut it out of your diet completely, at least moderate its intake as these two will irritate your bladder and aggravate your symptoms. Write this down on a sticky note and put it next to the walnut. Cut back at least 50% of your daily coffee and alcohol consumption.
4. Also, be moderate on usage of over-the-counter drugs and decongestants. Remember, whatever drugs you use must come out through urination, unless you know of another way that we are not privy to. Certain drugs cause the muscles that control urine flow from your urethral sphincter to tighten. Drink a bit of vinegar with your water daily and increase it by months. Here is another note that you should put on a sticky note: Eat your salads with oil and vinegar, not with salad dressings. I have added this to my diet and it has done wonders.
5. Exercise, I am sure, is not the word that you wanted to read in this book, but exercise equals retaining more urine and becoming physically fit, which will ease urination problems.
6. I don't know about you or the environment that you are living in, but I like warm weather near the ocean. I can tolerate cold, but prefer not to. It turns out that cold weather can

lead to urine retention and causes you to use the bathroom more. So, stay warm.

Determining How Far the Cancer Has Spread

Once a cancer diagnosis has been made via three separate opinions, you may need further tests to determine if or how far the cancer has spread. Many times the doctor will require you taking additional tests, which is a good thing, as you must be sure that it has not spread. Do not be in the group of men that do not require additional studies and can directly proceed with treatment based on the characteristics of their tumors and the results of their pre-biopsy PSA tests.

I personally took all five tests below, as I needed to have a peace of mind, what about you?

- **Bone scan.** A bone scan process takes a picture of your skeleton in order to determine whether cancer has spread to the bone. Prostate cancer can spread to any bones in your body, not just those closest to your prostate, such as your pelvis or lower spine.
- **Ultrasound.** Ultrasounds not only can help indicate if cancer is present, but may also reveal whether the disease has spread to nearby tissues.
- **Computerized Tomography (CT) scans.** A CT scan produces cross-sectional images of your body. CT scans can identify enlarged lymph nodes or abnormalities in other organs, but they can't determine whether

these problems are due to cancer. Therefore, CT scans are most useful when combined with other tests.

- **Magnetic resonance imaging (MRI).** This type of imaging produces detailed, cross-sectional images of your body using magnets and radio waves. An MRI can help detect evidence of the possible spread of cancer to lymph nodes and bones.
- **Lymph node biopsy.** If enlarged lymph nodes are found by a CT scan or a MRI, a lymph node biopsy can determine whether cancer has spread or not. During the procedure, some of the nodes near your prostate are removed and examined under a microscope to determine if cancerous cells are present.

Gleason Scores

Gleason scores are used to grade the seriousness and aggressiveness of the cancer.

When a biopsy confirms the presence of cancer, the next step, called grading it, is to determine how aggressive the cancer is. The tissue samples are studied, and the cancer cells are compared with healthy prostate cells. The uglier or different the cancer cells are from the healthy cells, the more aggressive the cancer and the more likely it is to spread quickly. What do I mean by "different cancer cells"?

Cancer cells may vary in shape and size. Some cells may be aggressive, while others aren't. The pathologist identifies the two most aggressive types of cancer cells when assigning a grade.

The most common cancer grading scale runs from 1 to 5, with 1 being the least aggressive form of cancer. Known as Gleason scores, these numbers may be helpful in determining which treatment option is best for you. The Gleason score adds the grades of the two most aggressive types of cancer cells; therefore, scoring may range from 2 (nonaggressive cancer) to 10 (very aggressive cancer).

Mine was an eight, and later, after getting three opinions, it was changed to zero, with no thanks to the four pathologists in Torrance and Culver City, California, who confirmed the Gleason score of eight. Pathologist Jonathan Epstein of John Hopkins Clinic detected their mistake.

Staging

After the level of aggressiveness of your prostate cancer is known, the next step, called staging, determines if or how far the cancer has spread. Your cancer is assigned one of four stages based on how far it has spread.

- **Stage I.** signifies very early cancer that's confined to a microscopic area that your doctor can't feel.
- **Stage II.** Your cancer can be felt, but it remains confined to your prostate gland.
- **Stage III.** Your cancer has spread beyond the prostate to the seminal vesicles or other nearby tissues.
- **Stage IV.** Your cancer has spread to lymph nodes, bones, lungs, or other organs.

Three typical types of prostate cancer complications include:

1. **Spread of cancer.** Prostate cancer can spread to nearby organs and bones and can be life threatening.

2. **Pain.** Although early-stage prostate cancer typically isn't painful, once it spreads to bones, it may produce pain, which can be intense. Treatments directed at shrinking the cancer often can produce significant pain relief. The treatments include hormone therapy, radiation therapy, and chemotherapy. If these treatments aren't successful, or while waiting for them to work, pain management with medications is an option.

   Not all people with cancer that has spread to bones have pain. Pain can be controlled, and there's no reason a person has to suffer with intense pain. If your doctor is unable to control your pain effectively, you may need to consult a pain specialist. This is not an area that I did any research on.

3. **Erectile dysfunction (ED) or impotence.** Like incontinence, ED can be a result of prostate cancer or its treatment, including surgery, radiation, or hormone therapy. Medications and vacuum devices that assist in achieving erection are available to treat ED. If other treatments fail, penile implants can be inserted surgically to help create an erection.

Why it is Important to Look at the Walnuts Daily.

For many men, a diagnosis of prostate cancer is frightening, not only because of the threat to their lives, but because of the threat to their sexuality. In fact, the possible consequences of treatment for prostate cancer, which include bladder control problems and ED, are a great concern for most men. Those two were certainly my major two issues while I was considering my treatment options.

Paying attention to high priorities in life and switch them around sometimes is difficult or next to impossible. When you bought those walnuts in the grocery store and placed them around, the idea was to constantly remind yourself to pay attention to your condition. I know that you have a ton of things on your plate, but enough time must be allocated to this so that you will still be around to enjoy life and pick up that same ton of those things. You would need to learn time management since you will have constant reminder of your health issue by looking at the walnuts throughout the day. Yes, I know, you do not have the time, but you have to make the time.

We will get into the types of treatments in chapter 7, which will be much more detailed, but for now, I like to start with some appetizers. Are you ready?

When I interviewed my uncle, who has prostate cancer and is currently under hormone therapy, he chose to do what nearly 95 % of prostate cancer patients chose to do: follow his doctor's recommendations for the method of treatment specific to diagnosis. My Uncle neglected to adhere to one simple rule: specific treatments recommended by a specialist may not work for everyone. If your doctor has treated many of his patients with hormone therapy, it does not mean that it is the only option for you, or that it will work for you. It simply means that he experienced success with this recommendation. When you have prostate cancer, male sex hormones (androgens) can stimulate the growth of cancer cells. The main type of androgen is testosterone. Hormone therapy either uses drugs to try to stop your body from producing male sex hormones or involves surgery to remove your testicles, which produce most of your testosterone. This type of therapy can also block hormones from getting into cancer cells. Sometimes doctors use a combination of drugs to achieve both.

In most men with advanced prostate cancer, this form of treatment is effective in helping to slow the growth of tumors. The idea here is that because it's effective at shrinking tumors, doctors use hormone therapy, often in combination with radiation, and sometimes with surgery. The therapy has revealed that hormones shrink large tumors so that surgery or radiation can remove or destroy them more easily. After these treatments, the drugs can inhibit the growth of stray cells left behind. Because most testosterone is produced in your testicles, surgical removal of your testicles or castration also can be an effective form of therapy, especially for advanced prostate cancer.

Some drugs used in hormone therapy decrease your body's production of testosterone. The hormones can set up a chemical blockade. This blockade prevents the testicles from receiving messages to make testosterone. Drugs typically are injected into a muscle or under your skin once every three or four months. What my uncle was not told was that with this type of treatment he might have to receive the drugs for a few months, a few years, and possibly for the rest of his life, depending on his situation.

The misconception that my uncle had, and certainly now you would not have, is that by simply depriving prostate cancer of testosterone doesn't kill all of the cancer cells. Within a few years, the cancer often learns to thrive without testosterone. Once this happens, hormone therapy is less likely to be effective.

Side effects of hormone therapy may include breast enlargement. I was surprised to recognize my uncle as he started to look more like my aunt with those large breasts and no bra. After the hormone therapy, expect reduced sex drive, impotence, hot flashes, weight gain, and reduction in muscle and bone mass. Some of these drugs can also cause nausea, diarrhea, fatigue and liver damage.

The surgical removal of your prostate gland must be the last option for you to take. It is called radical prostatectomy, which is another option to treat cancer that's confined to your prostate gland only. During this procedure, your surgeon uses special techniques to remove as much as possible from your prostate and local lymph nodes while trying to spare muscles and nerves that control urination and sexual function. I was scheduled for this surgery, but canceled a few days prior to the surgery date which I will explain later.

Although we will discuss surgery as the last option in chapter 8, let me introduce you to two surgical approaches available for a prostatectomy. One is called retro pubic surgery and the other perineal surgery.

1. **Retro pubic surgery.** In this approach, the gland is taken out through an incision in

your lower abdomen that typically runs from just below your navel to an inch above the base of your penis. It's the most commonly used form of prostate removal for two reasons. First, your surgeon can use the same incision to remove pelvic lymph nodes, which are tested to determine if the cancer has spread. Secondly, the procedure gives your surgeon good access to your prostate, making it easier to save the nerves that help control your bladder function and erections.

2. **Perineal surgery.** With the perineal approach, an incision is made between your anus and scrotum. There's generally less bleeding with perineal surgery, and recovery time may be shorter, especially if you're overweight. However, with this procedure, your surgeon isn't able to remove nearby lymph nodes.

The obvious choice from the above, as you can tell, is number one.

During the surgery, a catheter is inserted into your bladder through your penis to drain urine from the bladder during your recovery. The catheter will likely remain in place for one to two weeks after the surgery while the urinary tract heals.

After the catheter is removed, you'll likely experience some bladder control problems that may last for months. Most men eventually regain control. Many men experience stress incontinence, meaning they're unable to hold urine flow when their bladders are under increased pressure which happens when they sneeze, cough, laugh, or lift. In some men, major urinary leakage persists, and secondary surgical procedures may be needed in an attempt to correct the problem.

Impotence is another common side effect of radical prostatectomy because nerves on both sides of your prostate that control erections may be damaged or removed during surgery. Most men younger than age fifty who have nerve-sparing surgery are able to achieve normal erections afterward, and some men in their seventies are able to maintain normal sexual functioning. Men who had trouble achieving or maintaining an erection before surgery have a higher risk of being impotent after the surgery.

What about chemotherapy, you may ask. The misconception about this treatment is that chemo can cure prostate cancer. This is not the case. This type of treatment uses chemicals that destroy rapidly growing cancer, bad guys as well as healthy cells, or the good guys. Chemotherapy can be quite effective in partial treatment of prostate cancer, but it can't cure it. Because it has more side effects than hormone therapy does, chemotherapy often is reserved for men who have hormone-resistant prostate cancer.

While new chemotherapy drugs are being developed, current treatments are limited to a single-drug chemotherapy, multiple-drug chemotherapy and combination of chemotherapy and hormone therapy. The results of new drugs are promising, but extensive experiments are necessary. In the future, gene therapy, which we will discuss in chapter 9, will be more successful in treating metastasized tumors of the prostate. Current technology limits the use of these experimental treatments to a small number of centers that you must try to find in your area.

What is cryotherapy? That is when you stop crying

and start praying over your possible prostate cancer and then start a therapy. But seriously, this treatment is used to destroy cells by freezing them. Original attempts to treat prostate cancer with cryotherapy involved inserting a probe into the prostate through the skin between the rectum and the scrotum. Using a rectal microwave probe to monitor the procedure, the prostate is frozen in an attempt to destroy cancer cells. Poor precision in monitoring the extent of the freezing process often resulted in a frozen ice cream consistency and/or damage to tissue around the bladder with long-term complications such as injury to the rectum or the muscles that control urination.

Recently, smaller probes and more precise methods of monitoring the temperature in our behind and in and around the prostate have been developed. These advanced methods may decrease the complications associated with cryotherapy, making it a more effective treatment for prostate cancer.

Keep in mind that prostate cancer can't be prevented, but you can take measures to reduce your risk of getting it or to slow the disease's progression. The most important steps you can take to maintain prostate health and health in general are to eat well, keep physically active, and see your doctor regularly for the "the enjoyable finger test."

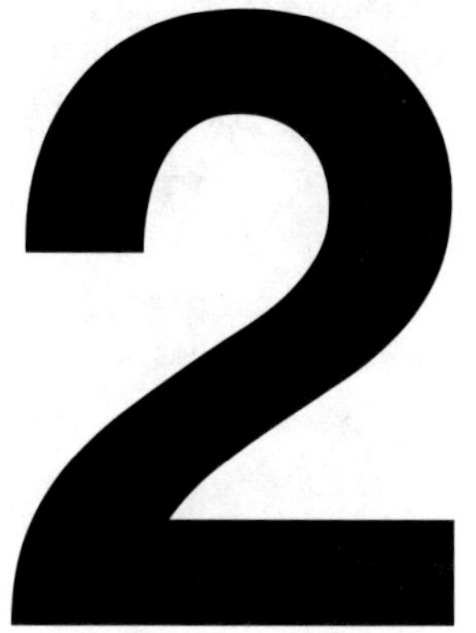

Chapter 2

Prostate Cancer Statistics and Diet.

One in six men will be diagnosed with prostate cancer and out of thirty-five men, one dies. More than two million men who have been diagnosed in the United States are still alive (American Cancer Society, 2007).

Other than the skin cancer, prostate cancer is the most common cancer. And behind lung cancer, it is the second leading cause of cancer death in American men. According to the American Cancer Society, the year 2008 brought nearly 187,000 new cases of prostate cancer, of which 29,000 died.

From ten men that are confirmed to have prostate cancer, nine are from the gland and regional stages such as bone (bone cancer). When compared to men the same age and race who do not have cancer (called relative survival), the five-year relative survival rate for these men is nearly 100 percent.

The five-year relative survival rate for men whose prostate cancers have already spread to distant parts of the body at the time of diagnosis is about 32 percent (American Cancer Society, 2007).

African American men have twice as much the mortality rate than Caucasian men.

According to a British medical journal, black men have a 300 percent more chance of having prostate cancer, and they must be diagnosed at least five year's earlier than white men in order to survive.

Between 1983 and 1990, 81.3 percent of Caucasian prostate cancer patients survived five years after the diagnosis. In the same period for African American cancer patients, the five-year percentage of survival was 66.4 percent.

Between 1992 and 1999, 98 percent of Caucasian prostate cancer patients survived five years after the diagnosis. In the same period, 93 percent of African American cancer patients survived five years after the diagnosis.

In 1998, the second leading cause of cancer deaths was in patients with prostate cancer. One hundred eighty-four thousand five hundred American men were diagnosed, and 39,200 lives were claimed. This record would be more accurate if we had disclosure laws in place that place in 1998.

Deaths from prostate cancer in 1999 in the United States were 31,729; that is 2,644 per month; or 610 per week (Society, 2007).

In the 2004 report of the American Medical Association:

1. Fifteen in every 1,000 men die within the first fifteen years after diagnosis of prostate cancer.
2. Forty-four in every 1,000 men die after the first fifteen years after the diagnosis of prostate cancer.
3. Twenty-four months is the median survival rate for prostate cancer patients with a high Gleason ranking at the time of diagnosis.
4. Two months is the median survival rate for prostate cancer patients with a high Gleason ranking who are still alive two years after diagnosis.
5. Thirty-four months is the median survival rate for prostate cancer patients with a high Gleason ranking who are still alive five years after the diagnosis.
6. There were 29,900 estimated deaths for prostate cancer in the U.S.

In Australia, between 1992 and 1997, 82 percent of Australian men between the ages twenty to seventy-four had a five-year survival rate after they were diagnosed with prostate cancer. Eighteen percent of the remainder lost their lives. In Australia, prostate cancer is taken very seriously down under.

- 2,852 men died from prostate cancer in Australia in 2002.
- Thirty-five men aged twenty to seventy-four

per 100,000 of the population died of prostate cancer in Australia in 2002

- In 2002, 4.1 percent of all male deaths were due to prostate cancer in Australia.
- Prostate cancer caused 2,665 male deaths in Australia in 2000.
- Prostate cancer accounted for 13.3% of male cancer deaths in Australia in 2000.
- Prostate cancer caused 35.9 male deaths per 100,000 of the population in Australia in 2000.

In England and Wales, between the periods of 1991 until 1995, the survival rate for prostate cancer patients between the ages of fifteen to ninety-nine years was 82 percent. That percentage decreased to 54 percent for men for a five-year survival rate. Between the ages fifteen to thirty-nine, the one-year survival rate increased to 78 percent, and it dropped to 46 percent for a five-year survival rate. Once the age group increased to forty to forty-nine, the one-year survival rate was at 83 percent and 40 percent for the five-year survival rate. Once the age group increased to fifty to fifty-nine, the one-year survival rate was at 88 percent and 58 percent for the five-year survival rate. So, as you can see, the survival rate percentage increased as the age increased.

In Canada, In 2004 4,200 men died from prostate cancer, according to Canadian Cancer Statistics from the National Cancer Institute of Canada.

Each year up to 2000, prostate cancer caused 245 deaths per 100,000 of the population for men over sixty-five in the U.S.

- Thirty per 100,000 Caucasian men died from prostate cancer between 1996 and 2000 in the U.S.
- Seventy-three per 100,000 African Americans died from prostate cancer between 1996 and 2000 in the U.S.
- Fourteen per 100,000 Asian and Pacific Islanders died from prostate cancer between 1996 and 2000 in the U.S.
- Twenty-two per 100,000 American Indian or Alaskans died from prostate cancer between 1996 and 2000 in the U.S.
- Twenty-four per 100,000 Hispanic and Latinos died from prostate cancer between 1996 and 2000 in the U.S.

Good Prostate Cancer Diet

You can't prevent prostate cancer, but what you eat can certainly affect the risk of you getting it.

Learn to love fruits and vegetables that you never liked, as what you never eat equates to the enzyme that you never had to build up your immune system. Your body can do a heck of a lot better with an equipped immune system. You have heard of chemical imbalance, right? Just imagine if every one of us had a perfect chemical balance, there would be little or no sickness. It is still not too late if you change your diet today. Stop the high-saturated fat food. Learn to eat broccoli, cabbage and other vegetables. A ten-year study conducted by researchers at the Harvard School of Public Health indicates that a high intake of cruciferous vegetables, such as broccoli and cabbage, may cut the risk of bladder cancer that could affect prostate cancer in men. Although eating plenty of fresh vegetables and fruits is important for overall health, only broccoli and cabbage seem to reduce the risk of getting bladder cancer. The Harvard doctors studied only men, and it's not known if the results apply to women.

High-fat diets have been linked to prostate cancer. Therefore, limiting your intake of high-fat foods and switching to fruits, vegetables, and whole fibers will help you reduce that risk. In this country, we are used to large portions of foods, and to prove that, just look at the portions of foods that you receive in the fast food places and restaurants. You must do everything you can to reduce the size of that belly, and as I mentioned earlier, the walnuts in your pocket and on your desk in your office must be constant reminders that you should just cut out the fat or the fat will simply cut you.

Foods rich in lycopenes, an antioxidant, also will help lower your prostate cancer risk. These foods include raw or cooked tomatoes, tomato products, grapefruit, and watermelon. Garlic and cruciferous vegetables such as arugula, bok choy, Brussels sprouts, and cauliflower also will help fight cancer.

Soy products contain isoflavones that seem to keep testosterone in check. Because prostate cancer feeds off testosterone, as we discussed earlier, isoflavones may reduce the risk and progression of the disease.

Are you a smoker? Vitamin E has shown promise in reducing the risk of prostate cancer among smokers. More research is needed to fully determine the extent of these benefits of vitamin E. If you are a smoker and you have been diagnosed three times with prostate cancer, I have a suggestion as to where you should put those cigarettes. No, not there, but at least place them next to the walnuts so you can feel the psychological effects.

Are you exercising at all? Are you really into exercise or do you prefer to watch exercise videos? Regular exercise can help prevent a heart attack and conditions such as high blood pressure and high cholesterol. When it comes to cancer, the data aren't as clear cut, but studies do indicate that regular exercise will reduce your cancer risk, including prostate cancer.

Exercise has been shown to strengthen our immune system, improve circulation, and speed digestion, all of which play a role in cancer prevention. Exercise also helps to prevent obesity, another potential risk factor for some types of cancer.

Regular exercise also minimizes your symptoms and reduces your risk of prostate gland enlargement, or BPH. Type A men who are physically active usually have less severe symptoms than type B men who get little or no exercise. Which type are you?

Let's assume that you have received three separate opinions from three independent doctors who based their conclusions on the results from different laboratories and all three opinions indicate that you do indeed have prostate cancer. What do you do now?

What I went through was a very typical reaction of any person receiving this sort of news. It was a feeling of disbelief, fear, anger, anxiety, emptiness, and depression. I soon had to learn that hiding the issue under the carpet did not diminish the fact that I had it, and the walnuts on my office desk were the constant reminder.

Now your supportive relatives and friends will come

forth to comfort you. They would say things like, "Oh, it is just a prostate cancer. Don't worry; it's not as bad as lung cancer or tumor in the brain. This is no big deal," and try to play it down. Remember, cancer is cancer, and although it does matter where it starts, it matters even more what stage it is in. And even though family and friends are extremely helpful in boosting your morale, what really makes a difference is your Faith. Reality is reality. Walking by faith and not by sight is the solution. This is the time that your faith is being tested, as mine was. You may not be able to get rid of these distressing feelings, but you can find positive ways to deal with them so that they do not dominate your life. The following strategies can help you cope with some of the difficulties of depressions caused by a true prostate cancer. They have helped me tremendously.

1. Remember how busy you were not being able to make it to church? Well, now you can. I can assure you that your family and money is important, but the uncertainty of what you have should occupy your mind. In my case, nearly 60 percent of my time was occupied with prayers, tests, doctor visits, research and related activities.
2. You should also think about joining a mini-church where people lay hands on you and pray for you. There is something mysterious about the power of prayer that can never be discounted.
3. Start to pay attention and highlight segments of this book that you can relate to, as

there has been a lot of research done that you may not be able to do alone.

4. Ask your three doctors questions and write notes, compile them, and read them from time to time. The fewer the surprises, the more quickly you'll adapt. Do not believe everything you read, as nothing is absolute.
5. Train your mind to accept that if it is what it is, there will be discomfort and a different style of living. Spend more time with your loved ones and get to know them better than ever before.
6. Keep your chin up. Fake it until you make it. Maintain your lifestyle routine as normal as you can. Don't let the cancer or side effects from treatment dominate your mind or day. You need activities that give you a sense of purpose, fulfillment, and meaning. But realize that initially you may have some limitations. Start slowly and gradually to build your level of endurance.
7. Do not let the devil into your mind via negative thoughts that could allow sad feelings. Seek diversions and plan at least one enjoyable experience every day. This might include pursuing something that you have never done before. Make it something you enjoy and look forward to doing it often.
8. How about building that gym that you always wanted or joining the gym? Get plenty of exercise. Exercise helps fight

depression and is a good way to relieve tension and aggression.

9. Open up to friends and strangers. Why not? There is nothing secret about you keeping what you have, and it is really not a private thing. You are much better off talking about it in public rather than keeping it a secret. You see, once you expose it, you will get exposed to plenty of experiences of others, extra help, and of course sympathies as well, but, at the end of the day you will know you are not alone.
10. You may find joining a support group helpful because it can provide you with a sense of belonging, giving you an opportunity to talk with people who understand your situation, and provide you with advice. Your doctor or someone you know who has experienced prostate cancer may be able to help you locate a support group. Or you can call a national cancer organization such as the American Cancer Society.
11. Are you leaking? I know, it is not a pleasant question, but are you? Well, it is diaper time. A rapid change of clothes during work is allowed. Getting used to this is not a big deal so long as you keep telling yourself that it is a temporary condition. And believe me, as you pray about the leakage, you will feel the difference. Your prayers must be focused on a specific issue.

12. Oh, my God, you now have impotence, and it is the end of the world, right? It is a new thing to learn about expressing your sexuality. Your natural reaction to impotence may be to avoid all sexual contact. Don't fall for this feeling. Touching, holding, hugging and caressing can become far more important to you and your wife. In fact, the closeness you develop in these actions can produce greater sexual intimacy than you've ever had before. There are many ways to make a night romantic. Learn what works best for you and your spouse.
13. Look for spirituality and grow emotionally. Stay tuned with your Creator. Your Creator knows the manual by which you were built. A nice Ferrari without the engine will never leave the garage. And a man without his spirit will never leave the bed. Your spirit can communicate with your Creator a heck of a lot better that you think it can.

Alternative Medicine and Acupuncture

Let's talk about all those nice-looking herbs in the nice shiny bottles that you see in health food stores; you can't resist buying them because the brand advertises prostate care: shrink your prostate over night, see results within 24 hours, and so forth. The marketing games can lead you to purchase products just for the sake of doing something about your symptoms (of course, your wife or girlfriend will see that you have done something about it). Once you take the pills for a few days without evident results, your wife or girlfriend may tell you that you have wasted your money. They are correct! 90 percent of the herbs that I bought were a waste of money.

Since herbs do not get regulated by the Food and Drug Administration, you never know what you are going to get. The side effects are another story.

It seems to amaze me that guys with BPH look for herbs that have saw palmetto as one of the ingredients to shrink prostate cancer. Well why not buy the pure saw palmetto tablets instead?

Saw palmetto or *Serenoa repens* is an exceptional herb; it is extracted from the ripened berries of the saw palmetto shrub.

Unlike other herbal supplements, it has been widely tested and shows much better results than any other herbs. However, it is important to know that if you have prostate cancer, it is too late to take this herb. Saw palmetto is recommended to treat the symptoms associated with benign prostate gland enlargement, not prostate cancer.

Saw palmetto is thought to work by preventing testosterone from breaking down into another form of the hormone associated with prostate tissue growth. In 1998, researchers with the Department of Veterans Affairs reviewed more than a dozen studies involving saw palmetto and concluded that the herb appears to be as effective as finasteride, the medication in Proscar, in reducing the size of an enlarged prostate. It also appears to produce fewer side effects. The researchers recommended additional studies to determine the appropriate daily dosage of the supplement and its long-term effectiveness.

Saw palmetto works slowly. Most men with BPH begin to see an improvement in their urinary symptoms within one to three years. If after three years you haven't noticed any benefit from it, it may not work for you. If you are raising your eye brows now, I agree, as I also have been told to take it for years, and I wonder if such statements are encouraged by the manufacturers. However, it appears safe to take saw palmetto indefinitely, but possible effects from long-term use are unknown.

One drawback of this herb, and many other such herbal products, is that it may suppress Prostate Specific Antigen (PSA) levels in your blood. This action can interfere with the effectiveness of the PSA test. That's why if you take saw palmetto or other herbal medicines, it's important to tell your doctor before having a PSA test. The results could be much worse for the risk of bleeding using anesthetics.

Try to figure that out. I personally have used saw palmetto, and I did not get any results. A recent study showed that it does not have any effects on symptoms. Typically, it is already too late once you find out that you have BPH, and from the interviews I had for this book, it appears that if one takes the saw palmetto for years, it will probably have some effects depending on the size of the prostate and how severe the growth is, but it is a tossup.

Frankly, I am not a pill type of person, and taking the usual vitamin pills is difficult enough to remember, let alone taking additional pills. Therefore, tablets were not a viable option for me.

While the medical world is vastly exploring options

of care that fall outside of the realm of traditional medicine, dietary supplements and herbal medicines continue to offer new ways to prevent or treat prostate disease and cancer in general. The question is, do these therapies work? Some are slowly gaining acceptance in mainstream medicine. But the benefits and risks of many products and practices remain unproven. Unfortunately, the production of these products is not well regulated, and the amount of active ingredients may vary from bottle to bottle or even pill to pill.

Here are a few herbal products that will help frequent urination or a weak urine flow:

- African plum tree (*Prunus africana*)
- African wild potato (*Hypoxis rooperi*)
- Pumpkin sides (*Cucurbita pepo*)
- Rye grass (*Secale cereale*)
- Stinging nettle (*Urtica dioica, Urtica urens*)

Taken in small to moderate amounts, these products appear to be safe. But they haven't been studied in large.

A few herbal and dietary products claim to help cure or prevent cancer. There's no scientific evidence that these products work, and some may be dangerous. Three popular cancer-fighting supplements include:

- **Chaparral.** Also known as creosote bush or greasewood, chaparral (*Larrea tridentata*) comes from a desert shrub found in the southwestern United States and Mexico. Research hasn't shown that the herb effectively treats cancer, and it can lead to irreversible liver failure.

- **PC-SPES.** This is an herbal mixture that has been marketed for treatment of prostate cancer. It contains eight herbs: daqing ye (*Isatis indigotica*), licorice (*Glycyrrhiza glabra, Glycyrrhiza uralensis*), san qi (*Panax pseudoginseng*), reishi mushroom (*Ganoderma lucidum*), Baikal skullcap (*Scutellaria baicalensis*), chrysanthemum (*Dendranthema morifolium*), dong ling cao (*Rabdosia rubescens*) and saw palmetto (*Serenoa repens*). A study of PC-SPES in the *New England Journal of Medicine* found that the product works like estrogen supplements. This herb reduces concentrations of testosterone that help fuel prostate cancer growth, and in some instances, may suppress the cancer, at least temporarily. However, the product commonly produces impotence and breast tenderness. It can also cause blood clots in deep leg veins and, if taken in large amounts, can be toxic. Another concern with this product is that it can mask the progression of your cancer. It reduces PSA levels, even when the cancer is advancing.
- **Shark cartilage.** Shark cartilage contains a protein that has some ability to inhibit the formation of new blood vessels within tumors in sharks. Shark cartilage therapy is based on the theory that capsules containing

> shark cartilage will do the same in humans and will stop and shrink cancerous tumors.

Another method of alternative medicine you might resort to is acupuncture; it is good for circulating your blood and energy through different points in your body, and it has been effective for a lot of diseases.

I took the treatment over ten sessions. If you decide to give it a try, you need to remember that one or two sessions is not sufficient, and once you start it, you must continue for at least fifteen to twenty sessions of up to thirty minutes, otherwise it is useless.

When you receive acupuncture as a therapy it is imperative that the practitioner is qualified. This is not about just finding a Chinese doctor who'd stick needles into your body; this is about your due diligence on checking the background and reputation of the practitioner who, by the way, doesn't have to be Chinese. Acupuncture practitioners are regulated by the Acupuncture Board and you need to make sure that his or her credentials are verifiable.

Here are a few things to take note of: make sure the needles come out of sterilized packages. Interview the practitioner about their background and experience. Be honest about your prostate cancer, and your fears. Before each treatment, ask where the needles going to be placed and if they will be heated through electrical current or some direct source of heat.

Though acupuncture is not a cure for prostate cancer, it can retard prostate growth.

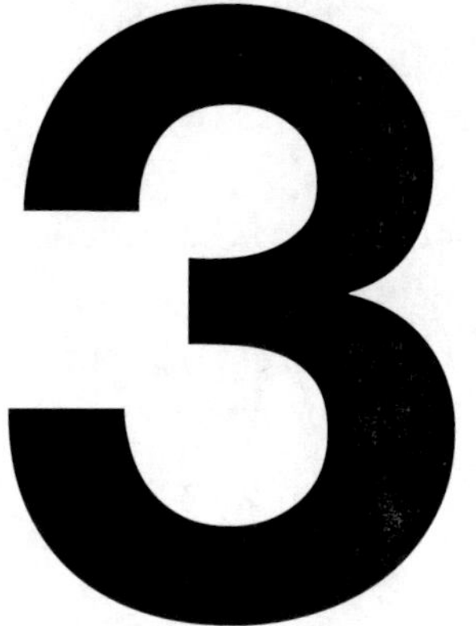

Chapter 3

Bladder Cancer

The reason I dedicate an entire chapter of this book to bladder cancer is the complications attributed to it which includes anemia, urinary incontinence, and a blockage of the ureters that prevents urine from draining normally into your bladder, but the most serious complication is the spread of cancer from the bladder to other organs, such as the prostate.

Two immediate and related concerns that directly attribute to a healthy or malignant prostate gland are bladder cancer and bone cancer related to your pelvis, as well as mate static cancer.

More than 90 percent of bladder cancer cases occur in people older than fifty-five, and 50 percent of cases occur in people older than seventy-three. Smoking is the greatest single risk factor for bladder cancer. Your exposure to certain toxic chemicals and drugs also makes you more likely to develop bladder cancer.

How does cancer develop in your bladder? That happens through a process controlled by DNA (the genetic material that contains the instructions for every chemical process in your body). When DNA is damaged, changes occur in these instructions. One result is that cells may begin to grow exponentially, eventually forming a tumor (a mass of malignant cells).

Your bladder is a temporary storage reservoir for your precious cargo, urine. It is located in the pelvic cavity. The size and shape of the bladder varies with the amount of urine it contains and pressure it receives from surrounding organs.

It is a triangle-shaped, hollow organ that is located in the lower abdomen. It is held in place by ligaments that are attached to other organs and the pelvic bones. The bladder's walls relax, expand, contract, and flatten to empty urine through the urethra. The typical healthy adult bladder can store up to two cups of urine for two to five hours.

This muscular balloon stores urine that your kidneys produce during the process of filtering your blood. Urine passes from your kidneys into your bladder through thin tubes called ureters and is eliminated from your body through another narrow tube, the urethra.

If we cut a cross section of the bladder and ureters, on the first layer we can see the inner lining of the urinary bladder, which is a mucous membrane of transitional epithelium that is continuous with that in the ureters. The second layer is composed of connective tissue with elastic fibers. The third layer is composed of smooth muscle.

Most bladder cancers begin in the specialized cells that line the walls of your bladder (transitional cells). The same type of cells occur in your kidneys, ureters, and urethra, where they may also give rise to malignant tumors.

Some cancer cells remain confined to the bladder lining. But other cancers are invasive, growing into or through the bladder wall, and eventually into nearby lymph nodes and adjacent organs. In time, cancer may spread (metastasize) to other organs, including your lungs, liver, or bones.

Bladder cancer affects men four times more often than women, and it occurs in Caucasians twice as often as in African Americans. Most people are over the age of fifty when they are diagnosed with this cancer.

If your urologist tries to explain what causes the bladder cancer, you can stop listening, as it is uncertain what causes it. However one thing is certain - if you are a smoker, you are helping the DNA damage that leads to cancer.

What caused me to stop smoking was comparing the cross section of healthy lungs versus a smoker's lungs in color. Just looking at that caused me to throw away the cigarettes. You may choose to continue to smoke until you get the bladder cancer and throw away the cigarettes then. Different strokes for different folks.

What causes the DNA damage that leads to bladder cancer isn't entirely clear. A very few cases show signs of inherited mutations, bladder cancer running in the family. More often, it appears that bladder-cancer-causing mutations develop during a person's lifetime. DNA damage may occur due to exposure to certain toxic chemicals, such as those found in cigarette smoke.

On the other hand, inherited factors such as how your body metabolizes certain chemicals may play a role. People whose bodies metabolize toxic chemicals quickly may be less susceptible to bladder cancer than are people who metabolize the same chemicals more slowly.

Although scientists aren't sure what causes bladder cancer, they've identified a number of factors that may contribute to its development, either by themselves or in combination with other factors. Because chemicals often exit the body through the bladder, many of these risk factors have to do with chemical exposure.

Although the actual reasons of why cancer within the internal organs grows faster or slower are unclear, you can change your diet and lifestyle to minimize your chances of getting cancer.

Being exposed to one or more of the risk factors listed below doesn't mean you'll develop bladder cancer, only that your risk may be increased. Knowing these factors may help you make changes that could reduce your risk.

- Firstly, are you a smoker? Smoking increases the risk of developing bladder, and obviously lung cancer by nearly 500 percent. I am assuming that most readers of this book are male. Statistically speaking, as many as 50 percent of all bladder cancers in males and 30 percent in females may be caused by cigarette smoke. I have no intention to convince you to stop today, but how about tomorrow?
- Secondly, what type of job do you have? Do you work in a chemical plant, shoe factory, aluminum, or leather-related product type

of environment? Are you a truck driver? Working in mining industry? Oil refinery worker? Well, that does not help you. You should not be around chemicals such as arylamine and carcinogens. And that is what we know as of now, which practically means not a lot. I have no intention to convince you to quit your job today, but how about the day after tomorrow?

- Thirdly, it is interesting that when the doctor prescribes radiation treatments, we do not think twice. "Oh, but that is what the doctor said." When I had to take the injection for the bone scan, I knew that such radiation would literally reduce and partially shut down my immune system for a while, but what were the choices? I agreed to it because it was a one-time deal, but what about the radiation and chemotherapy treatments? The radiation therapy of cervical cancer in women leads to an increased risk of developing transitional cell bladder cancer. The problem is that we are told only partial truth about the benefits of the radiation, but not the whole truth, as with Cytoxan, the drug that is used for chemo and how much it increases the chance for bladder cancer. No, I will not try to convince you not to take radiation or chemotherapy, but at least I warned you.
- Finally, the bladder infection issue. The short-term bladder infection is normal, but a long-term infection will increase the

chances of bladder cancer. I'd like to convince you that a bladder infection is not just another infection, but this is one infection that is internal, and you must be on top of it until it goes away.

There is no evidence that taking artificial sweeteners in your coffee and tea carries any risk of bladder cancer, although I think that the chemicals they contain cannot be good for you.

It is also a good idea to periodically examine your body for visual signs of potential problems. As you take your daily shower observe if there are any bumps, bruises or any signs of skin discoloration on your stomach or elsewhere. If you notice blood in your urine or anything unusual in the toilet, you must seek advice of your doctor immediately. By the way, taking urine samples right in your bathroom is just as good as in the doctor's bathroom. Investing in the sanitized sample containers is a good idea. Why? Because typically in the doctor's office you only have one shot, but in your bathroom, you have a heck of a lot more shots. We will not get into the details of how to take samples and delivery of such in this segment.

There are several types of bladder cancers, including the following:

- Transitional cell (urothelial) carcinoma. Transitional cell carcinoma is cancer that begins in the cells lining the bladder. Transitional cells also line the other parts of the urinary tract, including the kidneys, ureters, and urethra. Transitional cell carcinoma is the most common kind of bladder cancer, occurring in about 90 percent of cases.

- Squamous cell carcinoma. Squamous cell carcinoma is cancer that begins in squamous cells—thin, flat cells found in the tissue that forms the surface of the skin, the lining of the hollow organs of the body, and the passages of the respiratory and digestive tracts. About 4 percent of bladder cancers are squamous cell carcinomas.
- Adenocarcinoma. Adenocarcinoma is cancer that begins in the cells of glandular structures lining certain organs in the body and then spreads to the bladder. Common primary sites for adenocarcinomas include the lungs, pancreas, breasts, prostate, stomach, liver, and colon. Adenocarcinomas account for only about 2 percent of bladder cancers.

When bladder cancer is diagnosed, your physician will determine the grade and stage of the cancer.

Grade differentiates the cells from normal tissue and estimates the rate of cancer growth.

Stage indicates the extent the cancer has spread and if other body parts or organs are affected. The stage of cancer helps your doctor determine the best course of treatment and the outlook for your recovery. Additional tests may be needed to determine if bladder cancer is limited to the bladder or if it has spread.

The American Joint Committee on Cancer (AJCC) provides guidelines for staging of bladder cancer. The stages range from stage 0 to stage IV and have detailed criteria for tumor size, invasiveness, presence in lymph nodes, and whether or not the cancer has spread to other organs.

Bladder cancers are ranked based on how aggressive they are in a direct relationship with bladder tissues and tumors. How are these tumors classified?

- Stage 0–Noninvasive tumors that are only in the bladder lining
- Stage I–Tumor goes through the bladder lining, but does not reach the muscle layer of the bladder
- Stage II–Tumor goes into the muscle layer of the bladder
- Stage III–Tumor goes past the muscle layer into tissue surrounding the bladder
- Stage IV–Cancer has spread to lymph nodes in the area of the bladder

Let's talk about the case where the cancer spreads and which organs we must watch out for. In the order of importance, they are:

1. Prostate
2. Rectum
3. Ureters
4. Uterus
5. Lymph nodes
6. Bones
7. Liver
8. Lungs

How would you know if you have bladder cancer?

- Frequent visits to the bathroom
- Having lots of pain while you are urinating and incontinence
- Small portions of blood coming out with the urine
- Any tenderness or pain in the bones
- Losing weight rapidly
- Lots of pain in your abdomen

How is bladder cancer diagnosed?

In addition to a complete medical history and physical examination, diagnostic procedures for bladder cancer may include the following:

- Our favorite rectal or vaginal examination, 'the enjoyable finger test'–the physician can check for the presence of tumors large enough to be felt.
- Computed tomography scan (also called a CT or CAT scan)–a diagnostic imaging procedure that uses a combination of X-rays and computer technology to produce cross-sectional images (often called slices), both horizontally and vertically, of the body. A CT scan shows detailed images of any part of the body, including the bones, muscles, fat and organs. CT scans are more detailed than general X-rays.
- Cystoscopy (also called cystourethroscopy)–an examination in which a scope, a

flexible tube and viewing device, is inserted through the urethra to examine the bladder and urinary tract for structural abnormalities or obstructions, such as tumors or stones. Samples of the bladder tissue may be removed through the cystoscope for examination under a microscope in the laboratory.

- Magnetic resonance imaging (MRI)–a diagnostic procedure that uses a combination of large magnets, radiofrequencies, and a computer to produce detailed images of organs and structures within the body.
- Intravenous pyelogram (IVP)–a series of X-rays of the kidney, ureters, and bladder with the injection of a contrast dye into the vein. This test is used to detect tumors, abnormalities, kidney stones, or any obstructions and to assess renal blood flow. It may also be used to rule out other diseases or check for the spread of the bladder cancer to other areas of the urinary tract.
- Laboratory tests–tests may be performed on the urine to check for blood, chemicals, bacteria, and cells. The urine may be examined microscopically or grown in culture to check for infection. Cancerous cells may be detected using the microscope.
- Bladder tumor marker studies–tests to determine cellular characteristics and markers or substances released by bladder cancer cells into the urine.

- Ultrasound (sonography) a diagnostic imaging technique that uses high frequency sound waves and a computer to create images of blood vessels, tissues, and organs. Ultrasounds are used to view internal organs as they function and to assess blood flow through various vessels.
- They can use PET scans! This is called Positron emission tomography (PET) in nuclear medicine, a procedure that measures the metabolic activity of cells. A PET scan may show areas of cancer that may not be seen on a CT scan or MRI scans.
- Bladder biopsy–a procedure in which tissue samples are removed (with a needle or during surgery) from the bladder for examination under a microscope to determine if cancer or other abnormal cells are present.
- Bone scan. This imaging test is used to determine whether cancer has spread to your bones or not. During the procedure, a small amount of a radioactive substance that collects in bone is injected into a vein in your arm. A special scanner then takes pictures of all your bones. The radioactive substance highlights areas of abnormal bone.
- Chest X-ray. This test may help detect cancer that has spread to your lungs, though not always necessary for bladder cancer diagnostic procedures.

What are the options once you've been diagnosed with bladder cancer?

In stage 0 and 1, where the tumor is in the bladder lining or between the bladder lining and the muscle layer:

Option 1) a surgery to remove the tumor without removing the rest of the bladder

Option 2) my least favorite option is chemotherapy directly to the bladder

In stage II and III, where the tumor has gone through the muscle of the bladder:

Option 1) Surgery to remove the entire bladder

Option 2) Surgery to remove only part of the bladder, followed by radiation and chemotherapy

Option 3) Chemotherapy to shrink the tumor before surgery

Option 4) a combination of chemotherapy and radiation

Most patients with stage IV tumors cannot be cured, and surgery is not appropriate. In these patients, chemotherapy is often considered as a way of prolongation and not a cure.

What about immunotherapy? So long as the medications cause your immune system to attack and kill the tumor cells, it is the best way. What type of medications, you ask? Bacille Calmette-Guerin or BCG is given through a catheter into the bladder, and it does not feel good when this happens. As in everything else, there are side effects, such as frequent, urgent, and painful urination, plus irritable bladder. But don't worry, since these side effects will disappear in less than a week.

If the side effects are different, such as nausea, itching, chills, and blood in urine, you should be on your way to your urologist.

What if your doctor prescribes that your bladder, in part or in whole, should be removed because you are in stage two, or possibly three, or in between?

Don't agree on the surgery date yet. Get another opinion! And a third one. Most insurance companies will cover the second opinion, but not necessarily the third one. The question is how far are you willing to go to save your bladder in case there have been mistakes in the diagnosis? After all, this organ is deep within, and you only have one bladder that we know of, unlike the kidneys or lungs.

Are you easily convinced? What would your reaction be if someone tells you, "Oh, come on, what difference does it makes in having two versus three opinions?" or "How much do you know about the medical profession to say that the two doctors' diagnoses might be wrong?"

The point here is that it is your body, and until you agree on the surgery, it is your duty and responsibility to get a minimum of three (not two) opinions. Removal of an organ, such as bladder, prostate, or any other, must be the last and final option.

In men, when the entire bladder is removed, prostate and seminal vehicles may be affected or removed as part of the procedure, and in this case you need to be more knowledgeable and prepared.

In women with 100 percent bladder removal, the urethra, uterus, and vaginal front wall are also removed.

Take an active role in the decisions affecting your medical care. Learn as much as you can about bladder cancer and the treatment options that exist. As part of this process, you may want to consider getting three opinions from different bladder cancer specialists, such as an urologist, medical oncologist, or urologic oncologist.

Specific treatment for bladder cancer will be determined by your physician based on:

- Your age, overall health, and medical history
- Extent of the disease
- Grade and stage of the cancer
- Your tolerance of specific medicines, procedures, or therapies
- Expectations for the course of the disease
- Your opinion or preference

About 80 percent of individuals with bladder cancer have superficial and noninvasive tumors. Treatment for these tumors is often very effective with an excellent prognosis. About 25 percent of bladder cancers invade deep into the bladder wall and muscle. There is a greater risk for metastasis into other tissues in these cases.

Depending on the extent, bladder cancers may be managed with a single therapy or combination of treatments described below.

There are three main surgical procedures used to treat bladder cancer:

1. **Transurethral resection (TUR).** This is often used to treat superficial bladder cancer. During TUR, your doctor inserts a cystoscope, an instrument with a special lens and fiber-optic lighting system, into your bladder through your urethra. The cancer is removed with a small wire loop, and any remaining cells are burned away with an electric current. In some cases, a high-energy laser may be used instead of the electric current. TUR itself causes few problems. You're likely to have some blood in your urine or pain when you urinate for a few days following the procedure.
2. **Segmental cystectomy.** This procedure may be an option when a tumor has invaded just one part of the bladder wall. It removes only the portion of the bladder that contains cancer cells. To "remove" the tumor, the surgeon makes an incision in your abdomen. General anesthesia is used, and you usually stay in the hospital for a week. The main side effect of this surgery is more frequent urination. Although the problem is often temporary, it may become permanent in some people. Please do not take the word "remove" literally, despite what the doctor says.
3. **Radical cystectomy.** Doctors may use this extensive operation for invasive bladder cancer or for superficial cancer that affects a large portion of the bladder. It involves removing

the entire bladder, as well as nearby lymph nodes and part of the urethra. In men, the prostate gland, seminal vesicles, which produce some of the fluid in semen, and a portion of the vas deferens, are also removed.

In the past, the vast majority of men became impotent after a radical cystectomy. Now, new surgical procedures may prevent this problem in a very select group of men. Still, removing the prostate gland and seminal vesicles means that semen is no longer produced, and sperm is not released during ejaculation. Bladder cancer usually occurs in men after the years of active reproduction, but some men who have a cystectomy early in life choose to bank their sperm before surgery. As to which bank they will deposit the little ones, it is up to them.

Radical cystectomy can be life altering, affecting not only your ability to urinate normally but also your sexuality. Immediately after your bladder is completely removed, your surgeon reconstructs your urinary system so that you can eliminate urine effectively. There are several options for bladder reconstruction. The best approach for you depends on a number of factors, including your overall health and the extent to which the cancer has spread. In all cases, the goal is to maintain your quality of life as much as possible. Some reconstructive procedures include:

- **Urinary conduit.** This is the simplest operation with the least risk of complications. It involves isolating a segment of your small intestine and attaching one end of it to your ureters. The other end is connected to an opening (called stoma) in your lower abdomen through which urine drains into a small bag. You wear the bag outside your body and empty it three or four times a day. In the evening you can use a larger bag that allows you to sleep through the night.
- **Catheterizable stoma.** This type of reconstruction eliminates the need for a bag. Instead, your surgeon fashions an interior pouch capable of holding three to four cups of urine. You drain the urine from the pouch several times a day using a catheter. Because the size of the pouch remains the same, you must also drain your urine during the night.
- **Neobladder.** During this complex reconstructive procedure, your surgeon literally recreates a bladder. This is accomplished by connecting the same type of internal pouch used in a catheterizable stoma to urethra. As a result, you're able to eliminate urine without having an external opening, although you may need to use a catheter inserted through your urethra. Neobladder reconstruction isn't an option if some or all of your urethra has

been removed, and it may lead to a number of complications, including scarring, internal urine leakage, and incontinence. It also affects the ability to have sexual intercourse.

There are few non-surgical treatments of bladder cancer.

1. Photodynamic therapy (PDT) is still futuristic as of the date of publishing this book.

   This two-part treatment helps destroy bladder cancer cells. Initially you receive an injection of a chemical that is taken up by cancer cells, but not by healthy ones. The cells containing the chemical are then exposed to light from a laser, which kills or severely damages them.

   PDT may produce serious side effects, such as chronic bladder infections, bladder shrinkage, and long-term sensitivity to sunlight. While promising, this therapy is only done at a limited number of centers and needs further study before it can be routinely recommended.

2. Radiation therapy, which, as you know, is not my favorite, uses high-energy rays to kill or shrink cancer cells. It's most often used after an operation to eliminate any remaining cancer cells. When surgical treatment isn't an option, radiation may sometimes be used instead, but it's much less effective than surgery.

   Internal or external radiation or combination of both may be used in the treatment of bladder cancer. With internal radiation, a radiation implant is placed into the bladder for a direct effect on cancer cells. External radiation uses a machine outside the body to direct rays at a broader area; it is usually performed as an outpatient procedure, with treatments occurring five days a week for five to seven weeks. Radiation therapy for bladder cancer will have side effects including nausea, vomiting, diarrhea, and urinary discomfort, and it will affect sexual function in both men and women.

You may find that you become tired during radiation therapy, especially during the last weeks of treatment. External radiation can also cause your skin to become red, tender, and itchy, just as if you had sunburn. Radiation may also cause bladder or bowel incontinence, impotence in men, and irritation of the rectum, leading to diarrhea. These side effects are usually temporary, but they could be long term.

3. Chemotherapy uses anticancer drugs to kill cancer cells. Chemotherapy may be given internally by placing the drugs directly in the bladder, called intravesical chemotherapy. It may also be given systemically to affect cancer cells throughout the body.

   Your doctor may suggest having chemotherapy after an operation to eliminate any remaining traces of cancer, but sometimes you may have it before a surgical procedure in an effort to spare your bladder.

   This treatment is commonly used after TUR to help prevent a very superficial cancer from recurring. You are likely to have intravesical therapy once a week for several weeks.

This isn't an option if cancer cells have penetrated deep into the bladder wall or spread to other organs. In that case, chemotherapy drugs are given intravenously so that they travel through your bloodstream to every part of your body. This treatment is given in several cycles, which gives your body a chance to recover between sessions.

Even so, the side effects of chemotherapy—hair loss, nausea, vomiting, and fatigue—can be severe. They occur because chemotherapy affects healthy cells as well, especially fast-growing cells in your digestive tract, hair, and bone marrow, as well as cancerous ones.

4. Biological therapy. Now we are talking!

   Biological therapy uses the body's own immune system to fight cancer. In one form of this therapy, a solution called Bacillus Calmette-Guerin (BCG) is placed in the bladder, where it stimulates the immune system to kill the cancer cells.

   Biological therapy stimulates your body's own immune system to fight cancer. It's usually used after TUR to help prevent superficial bladder cancer from recurring. BCG, a bacterium used in vaccines against tuberculosis, is the most commonly used immune stimulant. It binds to your bladder, where it triggers a response that inhibits the formation and growth of tumors. BCG is administered directly into your bladder using a small, flexible tube for two hours once a week. Treatment may last six or more weeks.

During treatment with BCG, you may have some bladder irritation or blood in your urine and feel as if you have the flu. Your doctor may suggest medication to help reduce some of these symptoms. If you have a persistent high fever greater than 101.5 F that doesn't respond to pain relievers, see your doctor promptly for treatment. This may indicate widespread infection of BCG, which can be serious.

Coping with Bladder Cancer

Living with cancer is never easy. When I was diagnosed on my birthday in 2008, it was initially devastating. With my persistence and research, it took me three months to find that I didn't have cancer after all. However my life during those three months turned into nightmare and my daily prayers were the only thing that kept me going each day. Dealing with the physical effects of bladder cancer and its treatments can be especially difficult. This is particularly true if you have a stoma or urostomy bag. You may wonder how the changes in your body will affect your normal activities, your relationships, and your sexuality.

It is not the end of the world. It may help to know that having a stoma or urostomy bag doesn't mean you can't be active or live a normal life. The bags are small, inconspicuous under clothing and shouldn't leak. You can work, travel, exercise, and even swim, but make sure no one is in the pool!

Although there are no easy answers for coping with bladder cancer, the following suggestions may help:

- **Find ways to make your life easier.** If you have problems with incontinence or need to change a urostomy bag, try to sit in the back of a movie theater, concert hall, or meeting room. That way, you're less conspicuous if you need to leave for the toilet. Sit in an aisle seat on an airplane or train. Allow for breaks when planning long trips, seminars, or excursions.
- **Share your concerns with others.** When you feel ready, consider talking to someone you trust about your concerns. This might be a friend, a family member, your doctor, a social worker, a pastor, or spiritual adviser. You may also find it helpful to talk to other people with bladder cancer. They can tell you how they've coped with problems similar to the ones you're facing.
- **Don't be afraid of intimacy.** Your natural reaction to changes in your body may be to avoid intimacy. Although it may not be easy, it's vitally important to discuss these feelings with your wife. You may also find it helpful to talk to a therapist, either on your own or together. Remember that you can express your sexuality in many ways. Touching, holding, hugging, and caressing may become far more important to you and your wife. In fact, the closeness you develop may produce greater intimacy than you've ever had. Try it.

Intimacy issues may be even harder to address if you're not currently in a committed relationship. You may worry that no one will ever find you attractive or desirable. That is nonsense, as no one is perfect.

Chapter

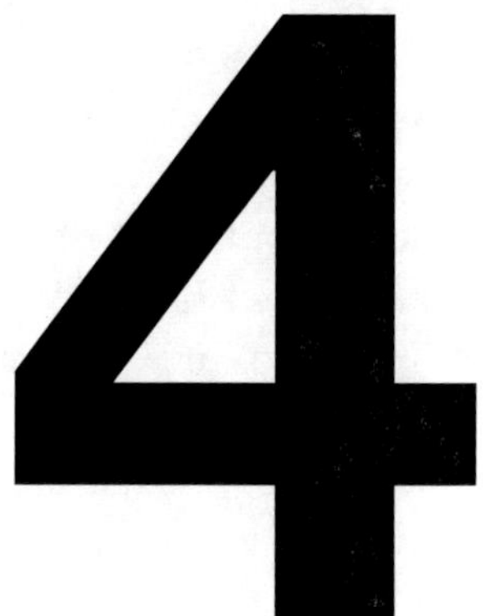

Prostate Cancer Metastasis to Bone.

There's no way to predict exactly how any type of cancer will spread, but, over the years, researchers have found that different types of cancers tend to spread in distinct patterns and that different types of cancer cells seem to prefer to settle in some areas more than others. For reasons that remain somewhat unclear, prostate cancer cells seem to prefer bone tissue and tend to migrate there after escaping the pelvic region. It would be great if we could throw a couple of pieces of bones and ask the cancer cells to eat them instead of our bones, but they have their preferences.

What is cancer in general? Cancer is a group of abnormal cells that grow more rapidly than normal cells and that refuse to die unless we shoot them one by one. Cancer cells also have the ability to invade and destroy normal tissues, either by growing directly into surrounding structures or after traveling to another part of your body through your bloodstream or lymph system. Microscopic cancer cells develop into small clusters that continue to grow, becoming more densely packed and hard.

Prostate cancer usually grows slowly and initially remains confined to the prostate gland, where it may not cause serious harm. But if left untreated, prostate cancer can begin to invade tissues and cause damage, and it may spread to others areas of your body, such as the pelvic bone, where it can cause significant harm.

Primary cases of bone cancer are relatively rare. Patients who develop bone cancer are more likely to develop the disease as a result of advanced prostate cancer metastasis. In prostate cancer, extension leading to bone disease is designated by a clinical stage. If a person develops bone disease as a result of prostate cancer, he does not have bone cancer. Because the cancer is classified according to where it originated, he has prostate cancer with bone metastasis.

Once the cells settle in, they're known as prostate cancer *bone metastases*. Unlike bone cancer, which originates in the bone, prostate cancer bone metastases are actually collections of prostate cancer cells that happen to be sitting within the bones. Therefore, the same treatments that are used to kill prostate cancer cells in other areas are often used in men with bone metastases as well.

Timely treatments are important because the prostate cancer cells in the bone don't just sit there idly. They interact with the bone tissue, often disrupting the normal growth and function of the bone and weakening it.

So in addition to any traditional anti-cancer treatments that your doctors might have already given you, treatment strategies for bone metastases also have to focus on making sure that your bones stay as healthy and strong as possible.

Symptoms of advanced prostate cancer bone metastases may cause stiffness or frequent soreness in areas such as the lower back, hips, and thighs. Some patients will experience more severe pain than others. As the disease progresses, some prostate cancer patients begin chemotherapy or external radiation therapy to alleviate the pain associated with bone cancer.

Most cases of prostate cancer, however, usually grow very slowly. Many men who have prostate cancer die from causes other than the cancer before their prostate cancer would have time to reach the advanced stage. The slow growth of the disease gives you an advantage and is one of the reasons why you should be observant to any symptoms mentioned here and constantly increase your knowledge about the disease. Regular testing to monitor the disease for sudden progression will save you from an invasive treatment.

Metastases are more likely to occur during advanced prostate cancer. Metastatic disease refers to prostate cancer that has left the prostate gland and its neighboring organs. Advanced prostate cancer bone metastasis and lymph node metastasis, which can be local or distant, are both associated with advanced prostate cancer.

If prostate cancer is detected early when it's still confined to the prostate gland, you have a better chance of successful treatment with no metastases and with minimal or short-term side effects. Successful treatment of cancer that has spread beyond the prostate gland is more difficult. But treatments exist that can help control prostate cancer.

Metastasis occurs through a process called angiogenesis. Angiogenesis is the process by which new blood vessels are formed; malignant cells are capable of "hitching a ride" into another part of the body. The malignant cells can commonly become lodged in the bones or lymph nodes. From there, the cells take root and start dividing uncontrollably.

Prostate cancer has a direct relationship to lymph node metastasis. The body produces fluid called lymph, which contains white blood cells and circulates through the lymphatic system. Lymph nodes are small oval or circular organs that filter this fluid. Cancerous cells that circulate through the body can become trapped in the lymph nodes. Once trapped, cancerous cells can begin their cycle of unhealthy division and result in lymph node metastasis.

There are two types of lymph node metastasis: local and distant. Two lymph nodes lie on either side of the bladder. Because these nodes are close to the prostate gland, metastasis is considered local. If cancerous cells begin to grow in any other lymph node, the metastasis is considered distant.

What causes prostate cancer and metastatic disease and why some types behave differently are unknown. Research suggests that a combination of factors may play a role, including heredity, ethnicity, hormones, diet, and the environment.

Knowing the risk factors for prostate cancer can help you determine if and when you want to begin prostate cancer screening. The main risk factors include:

- [Age.] As you age, your risk of prostate cancer increases. If you're fifty or older, you might want to see your doctor to discuss beginning of a routine prostate cancer screening. The American Cancer Society and the American Urological Association (AUA), recommend having an annual blood test to check for PSA beginning at age fifty, or earlier if you're at high risk for cancer. If you're African American or have a family history of the disease, you may want to begin at a younger age.
- [Race or ethnicity]. For reasons that aren't well understood, African American men have a higher risk of developing and dying of prostate cancer, about 500 percent, according to a British medical journal.
- [Diet and weight.] A high-fat diet and obesity may increase your risk of prostate cancer. Researchers theorize that fat increases production of the hormone testosterone, which may promote the development of prostate cancer cells.
- [Family history.] It is a no brainier that if a close family member such as your father or brother has prostate cancer; your risk of the disease is greater than that of the average American man. This must be disclosed to your urologist.
- [Testosterone levels.] High levels of testosterone in your body equals a greater chance of developing prostate cancer. Because tes-

tosterone naturally stimulates the growth of the prostate gland, men who have high levels of testosterone, such as men who use testosterone therapy, are more likely to develop prostate cancer than are men who have lower levels of testosterone. Long-term testosterone treatment could cause prostate gland enlargement. Also, you must be concerned that testosterone therapy might fuel the growth of prostate cancer that is already present. It is time to ask the question that relates to how active you are in sex. The more active you are, the more chance of BPH you have.

- [Medical history.] Surgery to become infertile or a vasectomy may or may not make a difference in developing BPH. There has been no conclusive evidence to support such research, and as of the date of publishing this book, research on this issue is ongoing.

Detecting and Managing Bone Metastases

As discussed earlier, prostate cancer often doesn't produce any symptoms in its early stages. That's why many cases of prostate cancer aren't detected until it has spread beyond the prostate. I certainly hope that by reading this book you will advise your friends and relatives to consider checkups even though there are no symptoms to point your finger at.

When prostate cancer cells spread outward, away from the prostate, prostate cancer cells tend to settle first locally, affecting the pelvic bone, the lower spine, and the upper thighs. You must learn to be sensitive to minor pain in your pelvis, the lower portion of your spine, and your thighs. You will experience pelvic area pain as a first sign that the cancer might have spread to the bone.

To review the symptoms of prostate cancer in a category related to possible bone cancer, see if you have any of the following signs:

- Dull pain in your lower pelvic area
- Urgency of urination
- Difficulty starting urination
- Pain during urination
- Weak urine flow and dribbling
- Intermittent urine flow
- A sensation that your bladder doesn't empty
- Frequent urination at night
- Blood in your urine
- Painful ejaculation
- General pain in your lower back, hips, or upper thighs
- Loss of appetite and weight
- Persistent bone pain

Once prostate cancer cells settle in the bone, they cause bone pain, fracture, or other complications that can significantly impair one's healthy bone structure.

The gold standard test for detection of the bone metastases is the bone scan. A radioactive substance that acts like a dye is injected in a vein, and images of the entire skeleton are taken. The dye-like material highlights areas where bone tissue is changing rapidly, a hallmark effect of prostate cancer bone metastases.

Bone scans can detect even small amounts of increased bone metabolism, but not all changes are caused by prostate cancer bone metastases. The dye might be detecting changes in the bone due to a previous fracture, infection, arthritis, or even bone loss that can result from the use of hormone therapy. A complete medical history can help doctors better assess the results of the bone scan and therefore determine the best treatment approach.

When prostate cancer reaches clinical stage T3 or T4, it classifies as an advanced prostate cancer with the tumor that has extended beyond the prostate gland and all the goodies like bone metastasis or lymph node metastasis.

What are the anticipating complications at this stage?

Treatment for prostate cancer bone metastases has three goals: firstly is to slow the disease progression. Secondly, to relieve pain, and finally, and perhaps most importantly, to avoid the complications that stem from the weakened bone caused by the metastases.

I know that first thing that comes to your mind is the bone fracturing or cracking, but hold on a minute. It is true that bones that are weakened by metastases are more prone to fracture, and because the metastases often grow around the lower back and upper legs, hip fractures tend to be most common. Vigilant monitoring for fractures usually is sufficient; less commonly, surgery might be considered to stabilize bones at risk. This procedure can improve the chances of not fracturing the bones, and therefore help to stave off other complications down the road.

The most significant complication from bone metastases is spinal cord compression. A weakening of vertebrae by prostate cancer bone metastasis can result in the bones of the spinal column collapsing one on top of the other, compressing the spinal cord housed within the bones, as well as the nerves that run out from it.

Cord compression associated with metastatic prostate cancer can cause severe nerve damage, and possibly paralysis, if not treated immediately. Therefore, additional medications, such as steroids, might be used for men at high risk for a spinal cord compression, and surgery to stabilize the weakened bones might be considered. MRI scans can also be used to better visualize the health of the spinal column and to detect early any problems that might occur.

The symptoms of spinal cord compression are often similar to those seen with many other medical problems. For example, because bone metastases typically occur around the lower back and upper legs, compression of the spinal cord at that point can cause back pain, leg pain or weakness, or loss of bladder or bowel control. It is therefore important to recognize and address any symptoms as soon as possible. The earlier new fractures or a spinal cord compression is detected, the easier it is to treat.

If you have been diagnosed to have bone metastases, it has advanced and, you believe that you are considered at risk, before you start thinking of possibly replacing your affected bones take a step back and get two other opinions. Do not jump to any conclusions yet.

Instead of you going wild and crazy thinking negative thoughts, stay positive until... Yes, you guessed that right! Until you have three separate opinions from three specialized physicians that use different labs and are experts in this area.

Do not worry! Unless you have three opinions from the experts indicating so, your prostate cancer has not advanced.

Chapter 5

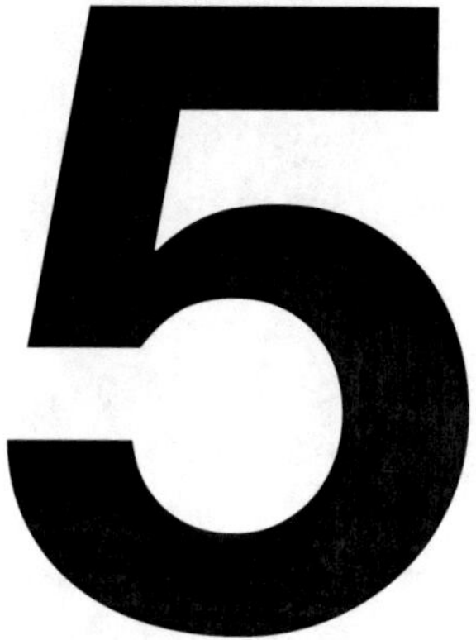

Prostate Cancer Tests, Biopsies and Diagnosis.

How old are you?

Were you told that your age must be fifty-plus before you could be a part of the group of prostate cancer candidates? Wrong. The best age to start the annual screening for prostate cancer is still up for discussion. If you are 40, you must have your PSA count determined. If it is too high (over 0.60 ng/ml.), then there is cause for concern. If it is an average score, then you need to monitor it annually to stay abreast of the prostate health.

A study presented at the 2007 meeting of the American Urological Association suggested that even a small increase in PSA in men ages forty-four to fifty may predict whether advanced prostate cancer would develop later in life.

Once you pass the age of fifty, and you are under seventy, and your PSA level is under 2.0, you must be screened every two years. The PSA test is not effective if you are over the age of seventy.

Do you have any family history of prostate cancer, such as your father, grandfather, uncle, or brother? Annual screening is a must.

You have to keep in mind a few things that will affect your PSA levels. You must not take the PSA test if you had sex within the last two days, since it can raise the PSA level.

At the same time, if you have BPH and associated treatments, they cause elevated PSA levels. Any surgical procedures or drug treatments for BPH, acute urinary retention, or a prostate biopsy will increase the PSA level.

Also prostate infection will automatically raise the PSA level. That is why the inflammation must be treated with antibiotics; otherwise the urologist may interpret the results of the PSA level as a predecessor to possible cancer.

When your urologist tells you that your PSA has risen to a range of 4 to 15 ng/ml, it is time to be concerned.

What is free PSA? You guessed it; it is free spirit. From your prostate, you have a small portion of PSA that leaks out into your blood stream. This is called free PSA, which is nothing but simple proteins. And it does not stick to other portions of proteins. It will circulate throughout your body, and unless you have cancer, it does not stick to other protein. If you have cancer, part of free PSA will stick, and in this case, there is less of the free PSA available in your blood stream. The test in this case is a ratio of free PSA to the total PSA.

The following results are used to determine if an elevated PSA level could mean cancer:

- A free-to-total PSA ratio of 20 percent or lower, with total PSA levels of 4 to 10 ng/ml, are suggestive of prostate cancer.
- A free-to-total PSA level of more than 20 percent, plus normal or even moderately elevated total PSA levels tend to indicate the presence of other, benign conditions, such as BPH.

What is a complexed PSA test? In this test, the circulating PSA bound to a molecule with a name of alpha antichymotrypsin. This represents nearly 90 percent of the total PSA in men, and it is higher in men with prostate cancer than men with just an enlarged prostate. This test, as of now, is controversial about its effectiveness. If your urologist suggests this test, I would think twice before taking it.

PSA tests alone cannot diagnose prostate cancer and used only as an indicator of a cancer possibility.

If the PSA blood test and/or the DRE (our famous 'enjoyable finger test'), reveal that you might have prostate cancer, and then your doctor will do a prostate biopsy to find out if the disease is present.

Ultrasound

An ultrasound procedure called transrectal ultrasonography (TRUS) provides a visual image of the prostate and is used if the finger test indicates the presence of cancer. An ultrasound is not effective as a diagnostic tool by itself because it cannot differentiate very well between benign inflammations and cancer, but the procedure may help to confirm an uncertain preliminary diagnosis and is useful as a guide for needle biopsies. Ultrasound enhancements, such as Doppler imaging or computer modeling techniques called artificial neural networks (ANN), may increase the accuracy of TRUS.

If the PSA tests indicate the suspicion of cancer, the biopsy is necessary. Your doctor or urologist is the one that performs the procedure in order to get samples of specimen, and it is sent to pathologists' laboratories. Practically all cases of prostate cancer must be diagnosed by removing a sample of tissue from your walnut and sending it to a pathologist that we hope and pray knows what he or she is doing. Most of this chapter is related to "what if the pathologist does NOT know what he or she is doing?" In my case, four pathologists failed.

Let's talk about what it takes to become a pathologist, as the pathologist's experience and training could make a large influence for the overdiagnosing or underdiagnosing of your prostate cancer. In my case, it was an overdiagnosis. When samples of your biopsy are given to the laboratory, typically you are not consulted as to which laboratory will be used, and 99 percent of the time, you are unaware of the pathologists that will be making opinions on your samples.

To be a pathologist, a medical graduate, a D.O. or M.D. must take at least five years of a residency-training program. Once that is completed, an exam must be passed through the American Board of Pathology. If the exam is passed, the pathologist becomes board-certified and is qualified for examining tissues or fluid removed from your body and rendering medical diagnoses. If the pathologist has not passed the test, the designation "board eligible" is given. Can someone tell me since when, a pathologist can fail the test and still become "board Eligible pathologist"?

The funny thing is that an M.D. and D.O. pathologist take the same exam, and there are no qualitative differences between the two.

I have a thought to promote an idea that an urologist must also take this exam. Why? Almost 95 percent of the time, urologists rely on the pathologist's reports without having to see the slides based on which those opinions have been made. You see, if your urologist had the same training and had passed the same exam, the possibility of a faulty report, like in my case, would be minimum.

Better yet, if in the future, it becomes a requirement for urologists to also be certified as a pathologist and the samples of your biopsy could be looked at in the urologist /pathologist lab, it would be phenomenal. It would be a perfect World if in all urologist's offices, the board-certified pathologist license credential was hanging on the wall, and the biopsy samples could be examined right then in their laboratory. In this case, every urologist is fully responsible for biopsy samples and opinions that come from his or her report, alleviating any possibilities of relying on outside pathologists. This still does not mean that just one opinion would be sufficient. The second and the third opinion would have to be obtained from other separate pathologists.

In such a perfect world, what would the pathologists do? Simple; reexamine the urologist opinion against the samples and confirm or deny the existence of the cancer. If such a perfect World ever becomes a reality, there would also have to be a "prostate cancer diagnosis recall program." What is that? Recalling faulty diagnosis or report, just like recalling defective cars, would be a requirement so that after a mistake was done, the patient is told the truth. "Sir, we are notifying you that despite the fact that your pathologist ranked your prostate cancer a Gleason 8 (which mine was), you really had no cancer. "Sir, we found that after removing and examining your prostate, you really did not have cancer." This kind of statements to victims could and would open lawsuits against the laboratories, pathologists, and hospitals, but it is the right and correct thing to do. Let the chips fall where they are supposed to but in the perfect World.

What is Prostate Biopsy anyway?

A biopsy is an internal pinching procedure in which several samples of body tissue are removed and then looked at under a microscope. A core needle biopsy is the main method used to diagnose prostate cancer. It is usually done by a urologist, with a surgeon's credential, who treats cancers of the genital and urinary tract, which includes the prostate gland.

The urologist inserts a needle through the wall of the rectum into the prostate gland. When pulled out, the needle removes a small cylinder of tissue, usually about half an inch long and one-sixteenth an inch across. This is repeated eight to eighteen times in each session, although most urologists will take about twelve samples. Then these samples are sent to the laboratory to see if cancer is present or not.

We will discuss such procedures in detail later, as I have repeatedly explained throughout this book that all the procedures that you are required to take related to prostate cancer must be repeated at least two other times. The first set of biopsies that I had was semi negative, meaning there was enough evidence there to take the second set. Being a firm believer in getting a second (and third) opinion, caused me not to panic at the first bad result, as I stuck to my motto "Check, double check, and triple check". This may not work for everyone as I will discuss later that certain biopsies are catastrophic.

Although the procedure sounds painful, it typically causes only a very brief, uncomfortable sensation because it is done with a special spring-loaded biopsy instrument. The device inserts and removes the needles in a fraction of a second. Most doctors who do the biopsy will numb the area first with local anesthetic. You might want to remind your doctor to do this, regardless of his or her plans.

Some doctors will do the biopsy through the perineum, the skin between the rectum and the scrotum. The doctor will place his or her finger in your rectum to feel the prostate and then insert the biopsy needle through a small incision in the skin of the perineum. The doctor will use a local anesthetic to numb the area.

Now, if you imagine the walnut-shaped prostate gland in your mind, the samples being taken will not really be from the entire 360 degrees of your walnut and the upper or lower portion. It is almost like random samples that may or may not be from the areas affected with cancer.

The biopsy itself takes about fifteen to twenty minutes and is usually done in the doctor's office. You will likely be given antibiotics to take before the biopsy and for a day or two after to reduce the risk of infection.

For a few days after the procedure, you may feel some soreness in the area and will likely notice blood in your urine. You may also have some light bleeding from your rectum. I also saw some blood in my semen, which lasted for several weeks after the biopsy.

Your biopsy samples will be sent to a pathology lab. There, a pathologist (a doctor who specializes in diagnosing disease in tissue samples) will see if there are cancer cells in your biopsy by looking at the samples under the microscope. From there, slides of pictures are taken. If cancer is present, the pathologist will also assign a grade. Getting the results usually takes up to three days, but it can take longer.

A patient I interviewed indicated that he developed prostatitis following a prostate biopsy which turned out negative for cancer but left him in severe pain. The second urologist diagnosed him having a possible bladder cancer and prescribed bladder biopsy and the results came out negative where Motrin was the only drug that he could use. Finally what worked for him was a series of "Prostate Messages" to take out the fluid that was formed.

Specimen processing

After the specimen is removed from the patient, it is processed in one or both of two ways:

1. Histologic sections. This involves preparation of stained, thin slices of less than five micrometers mounted on a glass slide, under a very thin pane of glass called a cover slip. There are two major techniques for preparation of histologic sections:
   a. Permanent sections. This technique gives the best quality of specimen for examination at the expense of time. The fresh specimen is immersed in a fluid called "fixative" for several hours. The fixative, typically formalin, which is a 10 percent solution of formalde-

hyde gas in buffered water, causes the proteins in the cells to denature and become hard and "fixed." Adequate fixation is probably the most important technical aspect of biopsy processing.

The fixed specimen is then placed in a machine that automatically goes through an elaborate overnight cycle that removes all the water from the specimen and replaces it with paraffin wax. The next morning, a technical professional, called a "histologic technician" or "histotech," removes the paraffin-impregnated specimen and embeds it in a larger block of molten paraffin. This is allowed to solidify by chilling and is set in a cutting machine, called a microtome. The histotech uses the microtome to cut thin sections of the paraffin block containing the biopsy specimen. These delicate sections are floated out on a water bath and picked up on a glass slide.

You may think that all of these are not important to you, but I disagree. What is important is the histologic technician's ability to cut thin sections and properly places them on the slides. In my second set of biopsy slides, this procedure was compromised.

Once the paraffin is dissolved from the tissue on the slid with a series of solvents, water is restored to the sections, and they are stained in a mixture of dyes. The most common dyes used are hematoxylin, a natural product of the heartwood of the logwood tree, *Haematoxylon campechianum*, which is native to Central America, and eosin, an artificial aniline dye. The stain combination casually referred to by pathologists as "H and E" yields pink, orange, and blue sections that make it easier for us to distinguish different parts of cells. Typically, the nucleus of cells stains dark blue, while the cytoplasm stains pink or orange. Also, in my second set of biopsies, the correct dye was not used and that caused misreading of cancer cells. And I was diagnosed with Gleason 8 by two laboratories and four pathologists. Once the mistake was recognized, the pathologists admitted that a wrong dye was used, which was their negligence. And if you think for a minute that this will not happen to you, you are dreaming.

b. Frozen sections. This technique allows one to examine histologic sections within a few minutes of removing the specimen from the patient, but the price paid is that the quality of the sections is not nearly as good as those of the permanent section. Still, a skilled pathologist and a knowledgeable surgeon can work together to use the frozen section's rapid availability to the patient's great benefit.

2. Smears. This procedure is not applicable to prostate biopsy, but it is good to know that it does exist. The specimen is a liquid or small solid chunks suspended in liquid. This material is smeared on a microscope slide and is either allowed to dry in air or is "fixed" by spraying or immersion in a liquid. The fixed smears are then stained, cover slipped, and examined under the microscope.

   Like the frozen section, smear preparations can be examined within a few minutes of the time the biopsy was obtained. This is especially useful when a radiologist uses an ultrasound or CT scan to find the area to be biopsied. He or she can make one "pass" with the needle and immediately give the specimen to the pathologist. The procedure can be terminated at that point, sparing the patient the discomfort and inconvenience of repeated sticks.

Pathologic Examination: Where Things Could Go Wrong.

1. The Gross Description

   The pathologist begins the examination of the specimen by dictating a description of the specimen as it looks to the naked eye. This is called "gross exam,". Some pathologists may refer to the gross exam as the "macroscopic." Most biopsies are small, nondescript bits of tissue, so the gross description is brief and serves mostly as a way to code which biopsy came from what area and to use for troubleshooting if there is a question of specimen mislabeling.

The last paragraph of the gross description gives the identifying codes of the slices of the specimen submitted for microscopic examination in cassettes. The microscope slides prepared from the processed samples will be labeled with the same numbers as the cassettes, and the pathologist doing the microscopic examination can, by referring to the typed gross description, know from what part of the specimen the tissue on the slide came.

2. The Microscopic Examination

   The microscopic description, or the "micro," is a narrative description of the findings gained from examination of the glass slides under the microscope. The micro is considered somewhat optional in a written report. In such a case, the diagnosis is done by the first and read and approved by the second pathologist. In my opinion there should at least be two or three pathologists looking at the same slides and consult with each other prior to such dictation of opinions. What looks one thing to a set of eyes will look different to another.

   The language of microscopy is much more arcane than that used for gross descriptions. It is way beyond the scope of this book to cover the nuances of descriptive microscopic pathology. In general, microscopic descriptions are communications between pathologists for referral and quality assurance purposes.

3. The Diagnosis

   This is analogous to the bottom line or a synopsis of a long financial report, which is my kind of report. The purpose of the gross examination, the processing of the tissue, and the microscopic examination is to build a logical argument toward a terse assessment of what significance the biopsy has in regard to the patient's health.

My first set of tests were sent to a pathology company in Torrance, California, and the second test was sent to a laboratory in Culver City, California, and all four pathologists there confirmed that I had a Gleason 8 (4+4), as I will explain it later.

I received a very friendly call from my urologist on my birthday that I should make an appointment to see him, because the results on the second set were positive.

That was not the present I expected to receive on my fifty-third birthday. I was told that yes, I did have prostate cancer. Moreover it was a high-grade cancer with a score of 8 based on the 1 to 10 Gleason chart and that it was confirmed by the two pathologists from the second lab in Culver City. My urologist said that this was a reputable lab he had dealt with for many years and that there was a very low possibility of error.

I was shocked. Why me? A typical question that anyone would ask, right? If you were the patient getting this kind of news, what would you do? I mean, it sounded convincing–two out of two reputable laboratories concluded that I had a prostate cancer and both came up with the same Gleason score result. It probably would convince most patients, but true to my belief of getting multiple opinions, I had questions buzzing in my head. What if there was a mistake either in sampling, delivery of the samples, mixing up the samples, or the pathologists were not looking at the right samples. The nightmare started to settle in. What if it was pure negligence? Even with a second opinion confirming the first one. I was still not convinced. You can call it gut feelings or sixth sense, but something did not jive. Listening to your wife and her instincts may need to be the next high priority.

Even with many samples, biopsies can still sometimes miss a cancer if none of the biopsy needles pass through affected area. This is known as a "false negative" result. If your doctor still strongly suspects prostate cancer (due to a very high PSA level, for example) a repeat biopsy may be needed.

My name was put on prayer lists of lots of my friends and associates. I had mixed feelings about help of prayers as I firmly believe in the power of prayer and have witnessed powerful healing others, at the same time my mind was telling me, "Are you kidding? You are two grades below cancer spread. Let's start to immediately to look for a treatment."

If you have been diagnosed, you need to have a thorough understanding of the Gleason grading system which is used to grade how far prostate tissue is from normal, healthy tissue. After the doctor has taken biopsy samples of your prostate tissue, the pathologist looks at the samples under a microscope and grades the tissue on a scale of 1 to 5. The low number, 1, is for cells that look almost normal (very slow growing cancer). The high number, 5, is for cells that are at least like normal prostate cells. Grades 2 to 4 fall in between.

Prostate cancer tumors often have areas of various grades. The pathologist identifies the two most prevalent grades. These are then added together to make the Gleason score, sum, or chart.

The Gleason score literally dictates how aggressive of a treatment you should take; in other words, you cannot think of minimum invasive treatment for a grade 8 or 9.

The first number is called "predominant grade" and represents over 51 percent of the samples. The second number must represent below 50 percent, but more than 5 percent of the samples. Remember that even 100 percent of the biopsy samples may not include the cancer cells.

A result may look like one of these:

5 is the combination of 3 + 2 or 2 + 3

Please note that 3 + 2 is totally different than 2 + 3. In the case of 3 + 2, the number 3 represents most of the cancer samples that is aggressive, with less of the samples that are less aggressive (2).

6 is the combination of 3 + 3
7 is the combination of 3 + 4 or 4 + 3
8 is the combination 4 + 4 or 3 + 5
9 is the combination 4 + 5 or 5 + 4

Because prostate cancers often have areas with different grades, a grade is assigned to the two areas that make up most of the cancer. These two grades are added together to yield the Gleason score between 2 and 10. The higher your Gleason score, the more likely it is that your cancer will grow and spread quickly.

In my case, a Gleason 4 + 4 meant that in two separate areas, I was just one tier below 100 percent cancer spread.

The reason why the Gleason grade and score are such key pieces of information for making treatment decisions, is because high-grade tumor cells, having lost the special structure, or "architecture," that made them work as part of the prostate gland, may not even put out much PSA.

I'd like to suggest that once your doctor receives a copy of your pathology report, you receive a copy of it as well and read it. The pathologist's report often contains other pieces of information that may give you a better idea of the scope of the cancer. These can include:

- The number of biopsy core samples that contain cancer (for example, "7 out of 12")
- The percentage of cancer in each of the cores
- Whether the cancer is on one side (left or right) or both sides of the prostate

Sometimes when the pathologists look at the prostate cells under the microscope, they don't look cancerous, but they're not quite normal either. These results are often reported as suspicious. They generally fall into two categories, either "prostatic intraepithelial neoplasia" (PIN) or "atypical small acinar proliferation" (ASAP).

What if it is PIN? The cells are basically still in place; they don't look like they've invaded into other parts of the prostate (like cancer cells would). PIN is often divided into low-grade and high-grade.

Men begin to develop low-grade PIN at an early age and do not necessarily develop prostate cancer. The importance of low-grade PIN in relation to prostate cancer is still unclear.

If a high-grade PIN is found in a biopsy; there is about a 20 percent chance that cancer may already be present somewhere else in the prostate gland. For this reason, doctors often watch men with high-grade PIN carefully and may advise a repeat prostate biopsy.

In ASAP, the cells look like they might be cancerous when viewed under the microscope, but there are too few of them to be sure. If ASAP is found, there's about a 40 to 50 percent chance that cancer is also present in the prostate, which is why I recommend getting a repeat biopsy and two other opinions within a few months.

It is important to understand your prostate pathology report. The surgical pathology report relays critical information about the biologic expression of the tumor. When tissue is removed from your body, it is sent to a pathologist, who examines it under a microscope and prepares a formal written report. Make sure to ask the laboratory for a copy of the report. And if they refuse, tell them that you will refuse to pay; it is your health and you have the right to have that information. It demonstrates your interest in being an active participant in the important decisions that you must make.

What should you look for in that report? A normal and a complete report of a needle biopsy should include:

1. Your name with your age, patient number, etc.
2. The accession number of the case (usually in the form of "S-year-number"). This number is very important, and it must correspond to

the number on the actual glass slides where your samples have been examined.

3. A gross description of the specimen, including the number and size of the tissue cores removed from your precious prostate and received by the laboratory.
4. The bottom line diagnosis, reduced to its most basic meaning of either benign (normal), atypical/suspicious, or malignant (cancer) with Gleason ranking.
5. The names and signatures of the responsible pathologists, along with the name, phone number, and address of the lab.

A schematic diagram of your prostate with the different biopsy locations identified will help you understand the location and distribution of your tumor. Remember that the biopsy core tissue represents only a small sampling of the entire prostate. As discussed before, it is common that tumors may be missed in a particular location or, even if sampled, may not be well represented by the tissue present in the biopsy report.

We will not discuss many benign conditions that mimic the appearance of prostate cancer.

A good pathologist mentions any findings he sees in prostatectomy, such as marked inflammation or signs of infection that may explain an elevated PSA. While such findings cannot prove that cancer is not present in an un sampled portion of the prostate, it might indicate that a trial with antibiotics for treating prostatitis should be attempted to lower the PSA value before a repeat biopsy is performed. Although the PSA level may rise as a direct result of the biopsy, it should decrease to baseline levels in four to six weeks. Remember that inflammations or signs of infections must not be there, as this is a false alarm that you want to turn off by taking antibiotics.

If a malignant diagnosis is made, it is imperative that a Gleason grade and score be assigned. The accurate assignment of Gleason grade is perhaps the single most useful factor in predicting prognosis and choice of treatment.

Small fragments of bowel lining are very common in needle core biopsies as the needle has to punch through this tissue to get to the prostate. The presence of a tumor surrounding a small nerve is a warning for probable extension of the tumor outside the prostate. This should be noted in the pathologists report.

The amount of tumor present is useful in estimating the total size of the tumor and may be used in formulas to predict the extent of the tumor found after possible prostatectomy. Tumor beyond the prostate is an important prognostic feature that should be commented on by a smart pathologist. If the pathologist has had experience, he or she can determine the gross chromosome abnormalities by merely looking at the routinely stained glass slide.

How honest should the pathologist be by swallowing his pride or letting go of his greed if he or she cannot determine or recognize the cancer's cells and faced with a choice of admitting the truth and sending the slides to another institution? Well, it is simple; he or she can simply pass any judgments and refer the slide elsewhere. It is a question of three elements: pride, greed, and experience. In my case, four pathologists thought that they could read the slides, and all four of them were wrong. As you review your biopsy report, you may see the phrase "Outside consultation," which should be a normal practice meaning that the pathologist recognized the case as difficult, and the slides must be sent to another institution for a second opinion or even third opinion. Do not expect your doctor to have read your report in full. You must read it over and over again in order to form a comprehensive understanding of the report findings.

Pathologic examination of any tissue in the setting of a potentially life-threatening disease, such as prostate cancer spreading to other organs, probably warrants a second and third opinion and expert review. Prostate cancer tissue poses an additional challenge of Gleason grading, which is done by visual determination. And in visual detection, there is lots of room for mistakes. For this reason, Gleason scores sometimes vary between pathologists.

What are re cuts? Re cuts are additional slides prepared from tissue remaining in the paraffin blocks. Re cuts are made either because a pathologist needs to see more tissue, "deeper in the block," to confirm or rule out a malignant diagnosis or because slides are to be sent to a different pathologist for a second or maybe third opinion. New tissue sections are cut, placed on glass slides, and stained. This entails extra expense to the lab, but dishonest labs will often absorb this cost rather than parting with their original slides. All opinions should be formed from information on the "original slides" and you must get involve as I did to make sure that the 2nd and 3rd opinions come from laboratories with original slides. It is your life, and your decision to leave it up to your doctor and pathologist to do, is a mistake. In my case, the re cut was sent as simply one slide, which showed how cooperative the pathologist was.

You must pay particular attention to any occurrence of such words as "atrophy," "atypical hyperplasia," "atypia," or "atypical glands" in the report, which indicate that the pathologist may have seen something abnormal in the specimen.

Other items of note that may appear on the report include the involvement of nerve twigs at the periphery of the gland, the size of tumor nodules with calculation of volumes, and the percentage of poorly differentiated tumors like Gleason pattern 4 and above within the tumor.

The ways in which the pathologist may help you is in the interpretation of laboratory tests such as free PSA, PSA velocity, and prostatic acid phosphates (PAP). He or she might also help to evaluate the different ultra-sensitive PSA tests that warn of early tumor recurrence and thereby provide the opportunity to initiate additional therapy when it would be most effective.

One of the most important pieces of information to be obtained from the post-operative pathology report is the assessment of surgical margins and capsular penetration. What is surgical margin? Organ confined tumor means the tumor is within the confines of the anatomical prostate. Established capsular penetration means that more than a few glands are found outside the normal confines of the prostate. When the surgeon removes the prostate, he often includes a thin rim of non prostatic soft tissue that surrounds the prostate. The outer aspect of this soft tissue constitutes the surgical margin.

One may take such information as the presence of capsular penetration and the status of surgical margins and combine it with Gleason grade and PSA to arrive at a probability that the cancer was not completely removed by surgery. Such a determination may suggest the early use of additional salvage treatments such as radiation and/or hormonal therapy.

Taking the time to understand your pathology and laboratory reports will teach you what you really have or do not have. Being active, learning and taking control, in my opinion, are more valuable than letting others dictate what you do or do not really have. I am going to try to explain certain aspects of the reports in different versions.

The Gleason score (GS) is a critical item; it is used as a variable in virtually every prognostic and treatment algorithm. An accurate GS mandates an expert pathology opinion.

An ideal pathology report will contain a description of each core sample that includes:

A. The location the sample was taken from (only available if the urologist puts each sample in a separate, labeled container)
B. A description of the core sample including length, diameter, and color
C. An indication of the type of any cancer found and the percent of the core that is cancer
D. An indication of the Gleason grades and the percent for each grade
E. An indication of perineural invasion, if present, which may be an indication of potential tumor spread outside the prostate
F. An indication of high-grade PIN, if present, which may be a precursor to prostate cancer

G. An indication of inflammation or prostatitis, if present, which may explain an elevated PSA and a low free-to-total percentage. This could be a precursor to PIN
H. Any other abnormal findings, such as atypia, atrophy, or BPH
I. The name and signature of the pathologist who reviewed the slides

If the pathology report is from a radical prostatectomy specimen, it should also include a description of the location, quantity, and extent of the cancer such as:

I. Cancer is confined to the prostate capsule
II. Cancer penetrates the capsule
III. Surgical margins are positive for cancer
IV. Cancer extends into seminal vesicles
V. Intravascular or intraductal involvement
VI. Cancer found in lymph nodes removed with the prostate

In summary, your pathology material may also include the biopsy material and/or radical prostatectomy specimen saved in the form of tissue blocks. As discussed before, the cancer tissue is placed into paraffin wax and stored as a tissue block. Such material is the source for glass slides that the pathologist uses to view the cancer material under the microscope.

You have all the rights to contact the laboratory that is involved with your pathology specimen, and make sure you know what their policy is regarding retention of this valuable resource. Many facilities will turn over the tissue blocks to the patient after obtaining a signed release.

Make the telephone call and find out. This could help you to enter future clinical trial and you do not want to be left behind.

Despite urologists' recommendations, I insisted on three sets of biopsies with a maximum number of samples using three separate labs and received copies of the reports.

Because a biopsy can miss very small cancer cells, sometimes three or even more biopsies are recommended if cancer is still suspected after negative results, such as when:

1. PSA levels are high. Two or more biopsies may be taken for high PSA levels. Even men with mildly elevated PSA (between 4 and 10 ng/mL) who test negative may be given a repeat biopsy. Whether a third biopsy is useful in these men if they still test negative after a second biopsy is uncertain, but in your case, is definitely certain, right?
2. DRE, or the 'enjoyable finger test', results are abnormal
3. Ultrasound results are abnormal
4. The initial biopsy yields microscopic findings that are suspicious
5. The initial biopsy detects precancerous cells known as high-grade prostatic PIN. No treatment is necessary with this finding, but these patients should be rechecked every three to six months for the next two years and then annually.

Your answer to the doctor's opinion of, "You have a prostate cancer," should be, "I do not believe it unless I get the 3rd opinion." As you can see, reading this book is placing you right in the middle of it.

After all, it is your life, not theirs. Are you willing to accept an opinion, even two opinions, when it comes down to being under the knife in the surgery room?

Yep, just a few cores of tissues and your impotence and leaky faucet depend on the correct recognition of these tissues. Yes, those funny-looking cells may or may not be cancer cells.

Chapter

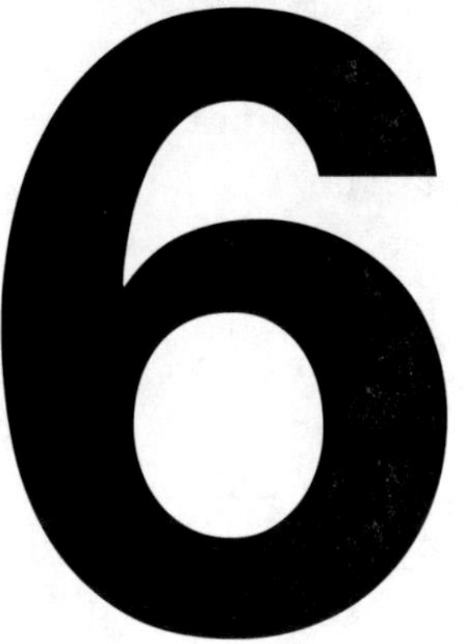

Wrong Types of Diagnoses for Prostate Cancer

The prostate biopsy can be a pathologist's worst nightmare as it is admittedly the most difficult among any other biopsies. And in case of a mistake, the pathologist's nightmare will become yours. Let's just hope that both you and your pathologist do not have the same nightmare at the same time on a same night.

If you think for a second that what your urologist tells you about your biopsy report is unquestionable reality and your urologist is 100 percent certain about it, you are wrong and do not hesitate to confront him or her. "Hey, what if it was your prostate? Would you be just as certain?" is what you should ask. Before starting to think about any cancer treatment, you want to be sure that the diagnosis is correct and accurate from three sets of urologists in three different geographic areas.

That is why you are reading this book, right? That certainly was my reason for writing this book. Getting a third opinion may seem unnecessary and a waste of time, but consider this: is it possible that the pathologist's report and diagnosis could be incorrect and incomplete? What if the report was issued for the right biopsy samples, but the samples were not yours, but someone else's? What if your name was typed on the pathology report, the report was correct, but it belonged to someone else? What if wrong dyes were used to recognize the cancer cells?, as it happened in my case and there are many more rooms for error.

Read what pathologist Jonathan Epstein, M.D. from John Hopkins Medical Center says about biopsies of prostate cancer.

"You are dealing with limited amount of tissue, and cancers tend to creep around the benign gland rather than forming as a solid mass. Imagine a Tootsie Roll, wrapped in paper. The cancer is like the paper, a veneer over an expanse of healthy tissue. And the veneer is often maddeningly ambiguous. So not only can the hollow-core biopsy needle overshoot and miss the cancer, the cancer cells do not match the pictures in the textbook. A pathologist will see something that he thinks could be cancer, but is not comfortable calling it cancer or likely over diagnose cancer. The next step is having a repeat biopsy, but in twenty percent of cases, the biopsy can miss cancer, so even it is negative, it does not mean that the patient doesn't have cancer. Looking at the Gleason grade based on a biopsy, and then comparing it to the actual specimen removed during surgery, and by and large, the Gleason grading that is performed, is disappointing."

As mentioned before, in my case, the two sets of biopsies were taken and sent to two different laboratories in southern California. Both reports from the laboratories, each with two pathologists, confirmed Gleason 8. In each set of the two biopsies within a month, the results were positive by both laboratories. I then made an appointment to be in John Hopkins Medical Center for the surgery. I was told that prior to such an appointment, my slides had to be sent for a final opinion. Dr. Epstein is the only pathologist that saw the original biopsy results and requested a new set of biopsy and then reversed the other four pathologists' previous positive reports and confirmed that there was no cancer.

What if the biopsy is labeled "atypical"? This diagnosis appears in about five percent of the biopsies reports at most institutions, according to Dr. Epstein. "Basically, what that means is that a pathologist will see something that he thinks could be cancer, but is not comfortable calling it cancer."

Another problem Dr. Epstein has found is that many pathologists seem just as likely to over diagnose cancer. "There are many mimickers of prostate cancer under the microscope, and people not as familiar with prostate biopsies can diagnose cancer when it's not." About one and a half percent of the patients who come to the Brady Urological Institute each year with a diagnosis of prostate cancer are found to have been misdiagnosed. "We switch the diagnosis. We say, 'This is not cancer, this is benign.'"

Perhaps the best option in the case of tricky diagnoses, according to Dr. Epstein, is to have the slides sent to an expert. About 70 to 80 percent of the time, it can be resolved as being definitively benign, which happened in my case. But even biopsies that seem straightforward deserve another look. "We recommend getting a second opinion before anybody undergoes any form of treatment," says Dr. Epstein. "It's just as important as getting a second opinion for surgery or radiation. You could have the best surgeon in the World, but if you don't have the right pathology, you could have the wrong thing done for you."

On this point, Dr. Epstein is blunt. "We have done numerous studies showing the reproducibility of Gleason scores in the general pathology community. By looking at the Gleason grade based on a biopsy and then comparing it to the actual specimen removed during surgery, we found that by and large, the Gleason grading that is performed is disappointing. All across the map, it doesn't correlate with what is seen in a radical prostatectomy. People have their decisions made—surgery or radiation or watchful waiting—based in part on a Gleason grade, when it's not accurate at all."

Beware of the low-grade Gleason score. Particularly erroneous, Dr. Epstein has found, are biopsies given low Gleason scores. "From the standpoint of patient care, the low-grade Gleason (a score of 2, 3, or 4) doesn't exist, and it gives a false sense of optimism. Even if I call something a 2 to 4 in a biopsy, when the prostate is removed in a radical prostatectomy, it will turn out to be Gleason 5, 6, or higher." Low-grade Gleason tumors do exist, Dr. Epstein says, "but where they exist is in the central transition zone of the prostate, not in the peripheral zone where you do biopsies. A low Gleason score is the kind of thing that shows up more in a transurethral resection of the prostate

(TURP)," a procedure used to treat prostate enlargement, in which tiny bits of tissue from the center of the prostate are chipped away and removed through the urethra. "If a tiny focus of low-grade cancer shows up on a TURP, it's not as worrisome as a tiny bit of intermediate tumor found on a biopsy. A low-grade Gleason score is valid on a TURP, but not on a needle."

In an effort to improve prostate cancer diagnosis, Dr. Epstein is teaching pathologists in a tutorial he devised for the Internet, a website for pathologists. "We just did it on our own," he explains, "because we think pathologists can do better than they have been. The key is education, not just getting frustrated." Epstein and colleagues have tried other approaches such as articles, he says, but have found that this website is "an amazing tool because it can reach so many people quickly." The online course—the first of its kind—take about an hour. First, pathologists are asked to grade a set of biopsies. Then, they're shown some of the telltale signs of various grades—Epstein calls them "tricks of grading"—and taught how to interpret another set of biopsies. Finally, they are asked to reevaluate the biopsies. "We've found that pathologists can make a dramatic improvement, just in this brief tutorial."

So the question that you could ask your pathologist, which is something I did not do, is very simple. "Would you consider signing up to this website and take the course?

As of now, a pathologist is the only physician who can make the actual diagnosis of prostate cancer, and I certainly hope that this practice will stop and yield to the practice of urologists passing the very same exam that the pathologists pass. Call it double insurance.

The reality is that sometimes mistakes are made in the diagnosis of prostate cancer. Diagnostic accuracy depends on the individual pathologist's training, experience, and judgment. In fact, a number of scientific articles have confirmed that such errors occur in cancer diagnosis in an average of 2 to 4 percent of cases. Based on these percentages, it has been calculated that 30,000 incorrect cancer diagnoses occur annually in the United States. And yours can be one of them. A great deal depends on the experience of the pathologist and his or her willingness to review difficult cases with other pathologists.

The American Cancer Society and the American Society of Clinical Pathologists recommend a second opinion for a cancer diagnosis, but I suggest a third opinion, as you want to know for sure it is what it is, don't you? The effort and expense necessary to obtain a consultation can be rewarded by the comfort of knowing that an original diagnosis was indeed correct.

Your rights:

A. You have the right to obtain a second opinion and check with your insurance carrier, as they may have to pay for it. Yes, I know the third one you need to pay, so write that check and sleep better tonight.
B. You have the right to select the pathologist who you want to review your microscopic (biopsy) slides or to ask your doctor to have your case reviewed by a pathologist who specializes in your disease. My recommendations here are to use the third pathologist outside of the state or the country that you

are living. My philosophy there is that maybe the first two pathologists received their credentials and training from the same facility and for this reason the third one must be outside of their area.

C. With your signed release, the primary pathologist must send your pathology material to the second and third opinion consultant of your choice.

D. The most practical way to obtain a second opinion is to not to talk to your oncologist or physician. I will not recommend any particular pathologist or laboratory in this book, but the third opinion should be based on a new set of biopsies and not the old ones.

E. While it is courteous to advise your doctor, you do not need your doctor's permission to obtain second and third opinions. But you will need to involve the doctor as the reference physician and pathologist who has your vital history and information in addition to the slides. That helps you get the best second opinion. Do not let your doctor talk you out of getting a third opinion or of sending the slides to the expert of his / her choice. A confident doctor will support your desire, as it is totally unorthodox and out of the box which matter here.

Pathologists' error rate is much greater than what you think.

American Cancer Society review of 226 prostate cancer tests from 2004 and 2005 found significant discrepancies requiring correction in 18 percent of the cases and that is not all.

Among the 18 percent, with significant discrepancies, they found six percent, of all those reviewed to be cancerous.

Of fourteen misdiagnosed cases, five patients reported problems, leading to a review of their biopsy and a correction in diagnosis, while the other nine weren't discovered.

The purpose of this review was to identify clinically significant errors, which is ultimately the purpose of me writing this book. The pathologists are humans, and the money and pride should not stop them from getting their mistakes corrected and informing the patients, as this does have an impact on the patient's lives.

Why can't we learn from the incident that happened in Wales England, as such mistakes are taken very seriously in Europe? We in the United States must have a much better checks and balances when it comes down to pathologists' errors.

In early 2008, hundreds of men from across Carmarthenshire in Wales, United Kingdom, waited a long time after it were revealed that there were mistakes made in their prostate cancer tests.

Carmarthenshire NHS Trust has sent letters to 528 patients who had prostate biopsies after tests revealed discrepancies.

It would take up to seven weeks for repeating the necessary tests to be made and some patients' diagnoses were recalled.

The trust has apologized and an information help line was set up immediately.

All of the men affected showed potentially cancerous markers in initial blood tests and were sent for a prostate biopsy, where the possible errors occurred.

Incidents proved life threatening, and as a precautionary measure, all 528 prostate biopsies carried out by the trust were referred to an external and independent agency for further analysis.

As a precaution, all results issued by the laboratory during this period were reexamined. The trust indicated that if mistakes had taken place, the numbers would be very small.

They also said some patients could have been given the all clear when they did, in fact, have prostate cancer.

Finally, the trust's chief executive made a statement. "The trust would like to publicly apologize for any distress this may have caused to the patients involved and to reassure them that the necessary steps are being taken to ensure that any errors are detected and dealt with as soon as possible."

The incident is the third in Wales and the second in Carmarthenshire. In the previous case, a pathologist at Llanelli's Prince Phillip Hospital was sacked after making mistakes in thirty-four examinations, resulting in ten patients being put on the wrong treatment regime.

The intention of pointing out mistakes and errors of pathologists in this book is not to scare you in any way from the pathologist that you have the report from, but to provide you the facts. I am sure, at some point, copies of this book could be sold to certain pathologists for dart practice, but nevertheless, a spade is a spade. Read on the percentages of mistakes in the followings institutions.

A 1999 study at Johns Hopkins University's School of Medicine found that eighty-six of 6,171 pathology reports, or 1.4 percent, contained errors serious enough to change the diagnosis. Even though 1.4 percent seem to be a low number, but eighty-six people's life was at stake and who can guarantee you won't be one of those eighty-six? These errors included mistakes in staging, misidentification of the type of cancer, and misdiagnosis of a benign tumor as malignant and vice versa. For example, prostate cancer staging and grading involved errors 20 percent of the time, skin cancer 2.9 percent, breast cancer 1.4 percent, lung cancer 0.6 percent, and female reproductive tract biopsies 5.1 percent.

A Dana Farber Cancer Institute study of 602 prostate cancer pathology reports found an error rate in the Gleason scores as high as 44 percent, with 10 percent of the pathology reports involving errors significant enough to affect treatment.

Yes, there are mistakes in other detection cases and screw-ups, for example:

- A study of ninety-seven bladder cancer patients at the Department of Urology at the University of Virginia Health Sciences Center found that second opinions resulted in significant discrepancies 18 percent of the time.
- A study at Ohio State University of 295 gynecologic oncology patients found changes of major clinical significance in 14 cases (4.7 percent).
- A study of 500 brain and spinal cord biopsy cases at the University of Texas Anderson

Cancer Center found that a second opinion resulted in a serious disagreement in 44 cases (8.8 percent).

- A study of sixty-six thyroid cancer patients at the Institute for Pathology at Leeds in England found that 18 percent had a different pathological diagnosis, with 7.5 percent resulting in a change in the management of the cancer.

A true story that cracked me up was in the news. In case you missed it, here it is. The dismissed pathologist at the center of a public inquiry into misdiagnosed medical tests in New Brunswick said "he's willing to apologize for any misdiagnosis mistakes, but is not willing to accept responsibility." Is this a typical pathologist mentality?

In an exclusive interview with CBC News Rajgopal Menon said he took "practically zero" responsibility for the incomplete tests and misdiagnoses at the Miramichi Regional Health Authority.

Menon, 73, worked as a pathologist at the health authority in eastern New Brunswick from 1995 until February 2007, when he was suspended following complaints about incomplete diagnoses and delayed lab results.

An independent audit of 227 cases of breast and prostate cancer biopsies from 2004 to 2005 found 18 percent had incomplete results and three percent had been misdiagnosed.

While testifying before the inquiry headed by Justice Paul Creaghan, Menon apologized to patients but said he was not aware of any errors in his work.

Menon told CBC News that if there were errors, there was a reason for it.

"I had a high volume. It's all volume related," Menon said. "If you have a high volume, you never catch up with your work."

Menon said hospital administrators have made him the scapegoat of a flawed system. He also suggested that racism might be connected to his removal from the hospital.

The former CEO of the Miramichi hospital, John Tucker, said he was "borderline desperate" for a pathologist when he hired Menon in the 1990s and didn't check his references closely. Do you think that this was an isolated case?

Further testing turned up more cases of people being told they did not have cancer when they did.

A peer review of Menon's work indicated the pathologist had serious medical problems, including cataracts and tremors in his hands, which could have affected the accuracy of his work.

College registrar Dr. Ed Schollenberg told the public commission that the first complaint about Menon was received in 2006. Menon was repeatedly told that if he retired, the matter would be considered resolved.

But you know what? There are many other pathologists like Mr. Menon out there, and guess what? You will never meet them. They are in their labs evaluating the biopsies and making mistakes left and right, just like the four of them in my case.

If I haven't convinced you by now about a good chance of pathologists' making mistakes, I have one more example for you. When the Canadian health officials have identified at least three prostate cancer patients who received wrong treatment after a senior pathologist made a mistake in their initial diagnostic tests, the cases were flagged.

Dr. Brock Wright, of no relation to me, the vice president and chief medical officer for the Winnipeg Regional Health Authority in Canada, said the latest findings of an investigation into errors made by the pathologist has so far turned up a total of seventeen cancer patients who may have received the wrong prognosis or treatment.

Wright said the three prostate cancer patients have already been contacted and were offered an immediate appointment with their physician to discuss further treatment. The three patients had their tumors in prostate gland removed, but further review of their biopsy found they may have needed radiation therapy after surgery. This means that the tumors were not 100 percent removed.

The pathologist was put on leave after an initial review of thirty-five of his recent cases revealed errors in 20 percent of them. Ten cases were flagged for discrepancies, including three instances in which patients suffering from cancer in their kidney and uterine area that died.

Wright said no errors were found in those three cases and patients died from terminal cancer, not diagnostic mistakes. But you know what? It could have gone the other way. It is such a close call. The difference between making money and reputation, take your choice.

In at least one other case, the pathologist failed to indicate that a patient did not have cancer in the lymphatic nodes on the patient's report. Wright said this was a serious error, but did not affect the patient's treatment or diagnosis. Well, to me if the pathologist failed to make a correct diagnosis in the lymphatic nodes, wouldn't that affect the treatment? It is one thing to take responsibility and admit the mistake and it is another to cover it up twice.

"In the pathology world, this is a serious issue," Wright said. Actions speak lauder than words, right?

Dr. Amin Kabani, a prostate cancer specialist and an authority involved in this case, stated that "Pathology is not an exact science, and complex cancer cases are interpreted by pathologists."

He also noted that "Typical error rates in pathology range between 0.5 and 14 percent and mistakes that affect a patient's diagnosis or treatment are rare, and occur in less than two percent of cases."

While Winnipeg health officials in Canada said, "Local labs are nearly fully staffed," Dr. Butany, president of the Canadian Association of Pathologists said, "Most laboratories in urban centers have been plagued by neglect and staff shortages for years."

He said, "Most labs are housed in hospital basements next to food and housekeeping services and haven't received much attention over the last decade, despite major layoffs and cutbacks in the early 1990s." Butany said, "Pathologists often work twelve-hour days, since the number of diagnostic tests and patients with cancer continue to increase," a combination that he said will eventually lead to errors.

"We are and we have been short of pathologists for several years," he said, noting a shortage of technologists who produce slides that pathologists review compounds the problem.

"Those who are there pick up the slack, and they work long hours on more complex cases."

Someone must tell Dr. Butany or others like him

looking for excuses, that it is best to tell the patients the truth in time, not years later, so that the patients know from the start that one, there are shortages of pathologists; two, pathologists are working twelve hours a day at a time; three, there is a greater supply of cancer biopsies to be performed than there are professional pathologists; and four, that there is a chance, however small, but still a chance that possible mistakes could take place, there is a choice to be made–choice to have another opinion.

Chapter

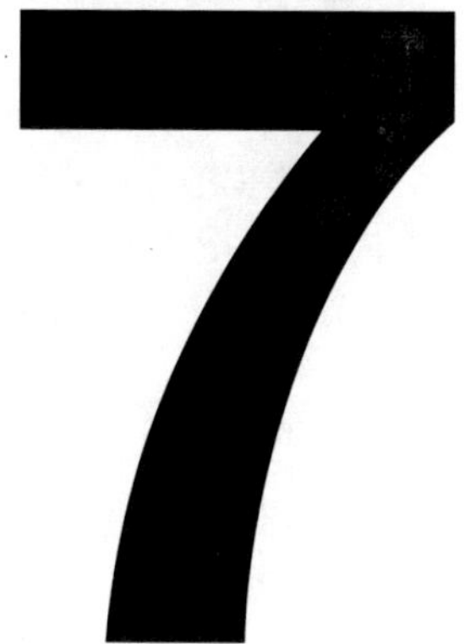

Medications and Treatments

No one likes to take medications. However, after prayers, they are the most common method for controlling moderate symptoms of prostate enlargement. You may be told that you need to take medications indefinitely, but that should be one out of three opinions. And that is why we will get into medications, side effects and treatments in this chapter.

Doctors use a variety of medications to treat prostate gland enlargement, let's dig into this.

- **Alpha blockers.** This stuff is pretty good for urinary flow and lowers the frequency of visits to your second office, I mean the bathroom. These drugs were originally developed to treat high blood pressure. They relax the muscles at the neck of your bladder, making it easier to urinate. So far the Food and Drug Administration (FDA) has approved four alpha blockers for prostate enlargement: terazosin (Hytrin), doxazosin (Cardura), tamsulosin (Flomax), and alfuzosin (Uroxatral).

Alpha blockers are quite effective for many men. The drugs work quickly. Within a day or two, most men notice an increase in urinary flow and a decrease in how often they need to urinate.

At present, we are not sure what could happen as far as the side effects, so take it easy and don't take a high dosage. Do not take the stuff with the drugs for impotence, as your blood pressure will go down.

- **Finasteride (Proscar, Propecia) and dutasteride (Avodart).** You would be given these guys only for the purpose of shrinking your walnut. I took them, but again, it boils down to whether you are a pill man or not. I am not, but I am taking Avodart in low dosage even now to maintain a constant shrinkage. These drugs relieve symptoms in a totally different manner than alpha blockers do. Instead of relaxing your muscles, they shrink your prostate gland. For some men with large prostates, the drug may produce a noticeable improvement in symptoms. It's generally not effective, though, if you have only a moderately enlarged or normal-sized prostate.

  Finasteride and the alpha blocker doxazosin together significantly reduce the risk of further prostate gland enlargement to the point where invasive surgery is not needed, depending on which stage you are in.

Finasteride takes a longer time to work than dutasteride. You may notice some improvement in urinary flow after three months, but for complete results, generally it takes up to a year. A small percentage of men who take finasteride experience impotence, decreased libido, and reduced semen release during ejaculation. But in most men, finasteride produces only slight side effects. The long-term side effects of this drug are unknown.

Finasteride has been shown to prevent or delay the onset of prostate cancer in men fifty-five years and older. However, finasteride also has been shown to adversely affect sexual function and to slightly raise the risk of developing higher grade prostate cancer.

- Nonsteroidal anti-inflammatory drugs (NSAIDs) might prevent prostate cancer. These drugs include ibuprofen (Advil, Motrin, others) and naproxen (Aleve). NSAIDs inhibit an enzyme called COX-2, which is found in prostate cancer cells. More studies are needed to confirm whether NSAID use actually results in lower rates of prostate cancer.

Taking certain drugs is dangerous as you see in the following real stories.

A physician prescribes neurontin and vicodin for a patient with intractable pain in urethra. It turned out that another doctor diagnosed him as having "parasite infection" and Flagyl was prescribed before running any tests.

He later notices that mucid discharge from his urethra. The third doctor prescribes azithromicion and doxycycline and that caused him flu symptoms such as chills, sweats and cramping of muscles. The fourth doctor diagnoses him as having prostatitis. This time Ciprofloxacin was given but did not work. The fifth doctor decides that he needs "prostate massage" and he must take Clindamycin. Severe pain in urinary tract starts following fatigue and short term memory loss. The sixth doctor after evaluation prescribes MRI and IVP Retrograde. MRI comes negative and IVP showed infection. This time IV Vancomycin 1000 mg was prescribed but did not do anything. Seventh doctor asks for HIV test which came negative. Number five doctor decides to put a catheter and instill Rimso 50/Unsyn. Again the burning sensation in urethra started. The same doctor drew blood for viral test. The number eight doctor after evaluation indicates that he has "active, positive stealth viral infection".

The above is an example of too many doctors with too many opinions and none were specialized. If the patient spent some times just to research and learn about his symptoms and would stick with three specialized opinion, none of the above would have happened.

Knowing about treatment options is essential. Non-surgical treatments and therapies are always more desirable because it takes care of the cause and not the symptoms and must be your first option to consider.

These therapies focus on enlarging your urethra, making it easier for the precious urine to come through the river.

There are several types of therapies available and may include the following:

- Heating or microwave therapy is the borderline between medications and invasive surgery. Transurethral microwave therapy (TUMT), which I call "Tum Tum," uses computer-controlled heat in the form of microwave energy to safely destroy the inner portion of the enlarged gland. It's more effective than medications for moderate to severe symptoms, as it was in my case, and it doesn't produce as many side effects as surgery. Heat therapy is often performed on an outpatient basis in the urologist clinic or hospital. Depending on the procedure, your doctor, and how quickly you're able to urinate on your own, you may need to stay in the hospital overnight. Heat therapy ordinarily requires you to wear a catheter for up to three weeks, but in my case it was only three days, and I did not enjoy the experience.

  The procedure could take up to half an hour. I was given a local anesthetic in order to ease the pain, but nevertheless, it was an uncomfortable half hour because of the high-temperature feeling inside of me and the urge to use the bathroom right there, during the procedure. I brought reading materials thinking I could kill two birds with one stone and get some work done during the procedure, but it was too uncomfortable to kill one of the birds. The microwaves emitted from the urethra antenna are aimed at the prostate inner tissues and induce oscillations of the water molecules, resulting in the release of kinetic energy, which generates heat. The follow-up study has only been up to four years in this therapy. No, I will not write another book in four years to tell you what happened.

The size and shape of an enlarged prostate is critical to the success of microwave therapy. If your prostate is very large or growing in an unusual shape into your bladder, this treatment generally isn't effective. The size is usually measured before in order to determine the success of this therapy.

The temperatures of over forty to forty-six degree centigrade could just barbecue the walnut, and for this reason barbecue sauce may be needed. During the procedure, a machine emits microwave energy through a urinary catheter. The catheter includes a tiny internal microwave antenna to deliver a dose of microwave energy that heats the enlarged cells and destroys them. Cool water circulates around the tip and sides of the antenna during the procedure to protect the urethra from the heat. Just make sure that the doctor takes out the antenna after the completion or you never know you may be transformed into a walking radio.

You will definitely feel the heat in the prostate and bladder area. You may also have bladder spasms. The response usually disappears after the treatment is finished. You can then go home and sleep and dream about the "hot dog on the stick" situation that you have had. Well, that is the real feeling.

It was my first time ever using a catheter and watching what was supposed to go to the toilet in the plastic bag mixed in with blood strapped to my leg. That turned me away from having an appetite. I must have called my urologist twice over the weekend on emergency, as I thought not only the tube to the catheter was coming out, but a lot more blood was visible. Well, nothing happened, as the tube typically is well placed. I saw him the following Monday to take the catheter out.

A few days after the procedure, I left the States with my family, and it took me several weeks before I began to see a noticeable improvement in my symptoms. I still did continue to see blood in my urine, but things were starting to get back to normal. And I was very satisfied with the procedure. Those who seem to respond best over time are men whose initial symptoms are mild.

It's normal to have urgent, frequent urination and small amounts of blood in your urine during recovery. There may be changes in the amount of semen you ejaculate, as I sometimes had little semen with blood. However, unlike more invasive surgery, Tum Tum generally doesn't produce impotence, incontinence, or retrograde ejaculation. With retrograde ejaculation, semen flows backward into the bladder during ejaculation instead of out through the penis and can result in infertility.

Tum Tum isn't recommended if you have a pacemaker or any metal implants.

- Cryoablation, which is cooling or freezing therapy for removing cancer cells. After many years of development, cryoablation is now being used to treat urological cancers, with far less risk and potential side effects than radical surgery. While it was initially developed for prostate cancer, its safety records and effectiveness have now expanded. The concept behind cryoablation is to create an ice ball within the prostate to achieve subfreezing temperatures—typically in the -40°C range—using argon gas. When the "lethal ice" temperature is reached, cancer cells, which are more susceptible to cold temperatures than normal, healthy cells, are killed and buried in your urine, and you may see the rascals coming out after the procedure.

Using the ultrasound monitoring, this procedure either can be in the outpatient area of a hospital or with just an overnight stay. Patients who have cyroablation procedures experience a rapid return to normal activities; have a much lower complication rate, and far less pain than those who have traditional radical surgery.

- **Radiofrequency therapy.** Transurethral needle ablation (TUNA), I call this one "TUNA fish," works by sending radio waves through needles that are inserted into your prostate gland, heating and destroying the tissue. As in Tum Tum, a special catheter is inserted through your urethra. The needles are inserted into your prostate by maneuvering the catheter. Now, just imagine if there were a radio near, could it pick up the frequencies and transmit it through your urethra?

  TUNA fish typically is less effective than traditional surgery in reducing symptoms and improving urine flow. Its long-term effectiveness also isn't known. Another drawback of the procedure is that it doesn't work as well in men with very large prostates. Side effects may include urine retention, blood in urine, painful urination, and a small risk of retrograde ejaculation.

- **High Intensity Focused Ultrasound or HIFU Therapy**. The HIFU procedure for prostate cancer therapy can cure the disease without the side effects of bladder control problems or erectile dysfunction that are common with surgical and other procedures. HIFU is a noninvasive, precise, and targeted procedure that reduces some of the risk of complications caused by traditional prostate cancer therapy involving surgery and radiation.

  HIFU is being used outside of the United States, as a therapeutic procedure for prostate cancer but check out http://www.pacificcoasturology.com/BenignProstate.htmBPH. The technology is not new to the United States, as it originated at the Indiana University School of Medicine in the 1970s and now, nearly four decades later, is going through the U.S. approval process of FDA.

  Since HIFU is not yet approved by the FDA for use in the United States, and it may take many years to stamp the procedure, it is technically considered as an investigational treatment. However, guess what? It is available throughout the world, including Japan, Europe, Central America, Canada, Mexico, the Bahamas, the Dominican Republic, and South Africa to name a few.

  When I was diagnosed with the Gleason 8, my out-of-country (and out-of-the-box) option was to take the trip to San Javier Hospital Marina in Puerto Vallarta, Mexico for an approximate cost of $25,000 and get it done. The trip was all arranged, but soon it was cancelled after I found out that there was no cancer.

What is HIFU and how it works? It makes me smile to think of so many different ways they have to come up to exterminate those little rascals that hide in our precious walnuts. They fry them, freeze them, zap them with a laser, whack them with radio frequency and television signals, and now they want to electro vaporize them. HIFU is transurethral electro vaporization of the prostate involves a special metal instrument that emits a high-frequency electrical current to cut and vaporize excess tissues while sealing off the remaining tissues to prevent bleeding. It sounds complicated, doesn't it? This procedure is especially useful for men at a higher risk of complications, including those who take a blood-thinning (anticoagulant) medication. Its long-term benefits aren't yet known.

- **Laser therapy**. It is getting better now. If none of the above is a good option, why not laser the heck out of the excess tissues in your walnut before we crack it up by a toaster? This procedure is performed similarly to other heat therapies, except it uses a laser instead of microwave energy, radio waves, or an electrical current to produce heat. It generally doesn't cause impotence or prolonged incontinence. However, some laser procedures require lengthy use of a catheter. Laser therapy includes transurethral evaporation of the prostate (TUEP), noncontact visual laser ablation of the prostate (VLAP), interstitial laser therapy, and photosensitive vaporization of the prostate (PVP).

TUEP is similar to HIFU. The difference is that your doctor destroys prostate tissue with laser energy instead of an electrical current. The procedure is generally safe and causes limited bleeding. It's often effective, with noticeable improvement in urine flow soon after the procedure. And guess what? The FDA approved this baby.

VLAP involves applying enough laser energy to dry up and destroy excess prostate cells. Because of swelling and prolonged sloughing off of the dead tissue, you're likely to retain urine for several days and will need to wear a catheter. You may also experience a burning sensation during urination for days to weeks.

Interstitial laser therapy directs laser energy inside the prostate growths rather than at the urethral surface. It safely and moderately increases the urinary flow rate and reduces the volume of the prostate. It also seems to work well among men with large prostates. Because of substantial tissue inflammation after treatment, you may need to use a catheter for up to three weeks. Uncomplicated urinary tract infections also are common. Interstitial laser therapy is a better option than surgery, especially if you have health complications. It doesn't cause any blood loss and uses a combination of local anesthesia and intravenous sedation to control pain during the procedure.

Photosensitive vaporization, or PVP, is a newer form of laser treatment for prostate gland enlargement. This procedure and its results are similar to transurethral resection of the prostate (TURP), which is the most common surgical treatment for an enlarged prostate. However, photosensitive vaporization uses laser energy instead of the electrical current used by TURP to destroy prostate tissue. In general, photosensitive vaporization is better for smaller prostates. PVP may also result in less bleeding and a shorter recovery time than with TURP.

- **Prostatic stents**. A prostatic stent is a tiny metal coil. The stent is inserted into your urethra to widen the urethra and keep it open. By golly, if you can't heat the walnut, cool it. If you can't use radio frequency or television signals, microwave it or stent it, and if all fails, shave the walnut, like they do it with "TURP". Tissue grows over the stent to hold it in place. This treatment causes little or no bleeding and doesn't require a catheter. It may be an option for you if you are unwilling or unable to take medications or are reluctant or unable to have surgery. Stents often aren't ideal for older men who have difficulty wearing or maintaining them or who are unable to tolerate the procedure.

  Some men find that the stents don't improve their symptoms. Others experience irritation when urinating or have frequent urinary tract infections.

> These complications, along with the high cost and potential difficulties in removing the stents, have reduced the popularity of this treatment. And bottom line, I do not recommend this procedure.

A drawback of the nonsurgical therapies is that no biopsies are done from your prostate gland, so you will not know if in fact you had cancer or not. During surgical treatments for an enlarged prostate, a small sample of your prostate generally is taken by your doctor and examined by a pathologist for possible cancer later, but in all nonsurgical treatments, this option is lost.

Chapter

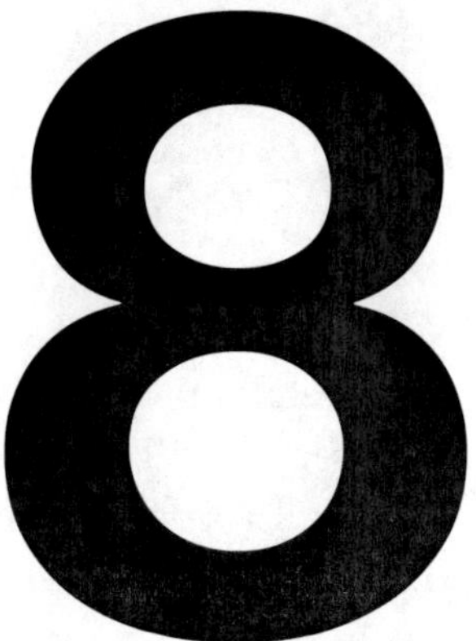

Surgery as the Last Option

Surgical and other similar procedures must be last on your list.

It is interesting that when you ask a stockbroker for real estate advice, you will get an inadequate or no advice at all. What sort of advice about nonsurgical treatments do you expect to hear from your doctor if s/he doesn't practice the minimum invasive or nonsurgical treatments or believes 100 % in radical surgery? Regardless, know that the answer you receive depends upon who you ask. Be very careful, as your life is more important than accepting and complying the surgeon's opinion.

When my second set of biopsy reports was generated, I made an appointment to show it to a top-ranking surgeon at the University of California in Irvine, and right away, after a short examination without any questions, I was ordered to schedule a surgery, the sooner, the better. I had already interviewed a patient that this doctor did the surgery on, a couple of years ago. After talking to him, he sounded like that he was satisfied with his decision of doing the surgery after his research. When I asked him about leakage and impotence, he tried to dodge the questions, but I inquired directly because I wanted to know if two years after the surgery if would I end up like him. When he noticed that I was getting too close to comfort, he refused to answer my simple but tough questions. I then met with his wife to ask those tough questions, and yes, I was right; the surgery was a mistake. After two years, there were still signs of impotence and leakage. How much of a research is enough? Are you happy with the research in this book? And have you done other research on your own? Are you researching the doctors and surgeons to get familiar with what they tell you? In addition on reading this book, are you researching to increase your knowledge?

At one time, surgery was the most common treatment for BPH and malignant prostate. But because of the increased use of medications and the development of other, less invasive therapies, surgery is on the decline. Today it's used mainly for more severe signs and symptoms or if you have complicating factors, such as:

- Frequent urinary tract infections
- Kidney damage from urinary retention
- Bleeding through the urethra
- Stones in the bladder
- High Gleason stages

When another prostate surgeon friend from Ontario, Canada found out that I made the schedule for the surgery with this doctor, he congratulated me, as he thought I made the right choice. Little did he know that I was simply keeping all my options open, as all options were going parallel until I dropped or exercised them? I made several surgery dates and had several biopsies scheduled until the very last moment at which time I decided whether to proceed as planned or cancel the surgery. Surgery is the most effective of all therapies for relieving symptoms of an enlarged prostate. It's the gold standard by which all other treatments are judged, and many doctors have extensive experience with it. However, it's also the most likely to produce side effects. Surgery isn't usually recommended unless it is absolutely necessary.

Surgery for an enlarged or malignant prostate requires a hospital stay. If you have surgery, you may need to take up to a month off work. You'll also need to avoid heavy lifting, jarring to your lower pelvic area, or straining of your lower abdominal muscles for up to two months.

The types of surgery for an enlarged prostate include:

- Transurethral resection of the prostate (TURP), which we discussed briefly before. I call it simply "shaving the heck off your walnut." This is the most common surgery for an enlarged prostate. During the procedure, you're given a general anesthesia or anesthetized from the waist down with a spinal block. A surgeon threads a narrow instrument (resectoscope) into your urethra and uses small cutting tools to scrape away or shave off excess prostate tissue. You can expect to stay in the hospital for one to three days after surgery. During your recovery, you'll have a urinary catheter in place for a few days.

When I interviewed my close friend that took the procedure, he said that although he was happy with the procedure, he wished he knew that the other minimum invasive therapies existed. He had done zero research, and just like others that I interviewed for this book, he trusted his doctor. TURP is effective and relieves symptoms quickly. Most men experience a stronger urine flow within a few days. You can expect some blood or small blood clots to appear in your urine afterward. Before you leave the hospital, you should be able to urinate on your own. At first, you may feel some pain or a sense of urgency when urine passes over the surgical area. This discomfort should gradually improve. In some cases, you may be sent home from the hospital with a catheter that is later removed in your doctor's office.

In some cases, TURP can cause impotence and loss of bladder control. Generally, these conditions are only temporary. Pelvic floor muscle exercises often help restore bladder control. Normal sexual function often returns within a few weeks to few months. However, it can take up to a year to make a full recovery from these side effects.

Another more common side effect of surgery is retrograde ejaculation. TURP may also produce scarring and narrowing in the urethra or bladder neck. This often can be remedied by stretching the scar tissue, done on an outpatient basis. Some men who have TURP may need some sort of prostate surgery again because the prostate grew back or the scar tissue from a previous procedure needs to be removed.

- **Transurethral incision of the prostate (TUIP).** This surgery is an option if you have only a moderately enlarged or small prostate gland. It's also an option for men who aren't good candidates for more invasive surgery for health reasons or because they don't want to risk sterility.

  Like TURP, TUIP involves special instruments that are inserted through the urethra. But instead of removing prostate tissue, the surgeon makes one or two small cuts in the prostate gland. The cuts help enlarge the opening of the urethra, making it easier to urinate.

  The procedure produces less risk of complications than other kinds of surgery. It doesn't require an overnight hospital stay, but it's less effective and often needs to be repeated. Some men experience only a small improvement in urinary flow.

- **Open prostatectomy.** It's called open because the surgeon opens you up and makes an incision in your lower abdomen to reach the prostate rather than going up through the urethra. During an open prostatectomy, only the inner portion of your prostate gland is removed, leaving the outer portion intact. This type of surgery is generally performed only if you have an excessively large prostate, bladder damage, or other complicating factors, such as bladder stones or urethral strictures.

Open prostatectomy poses the greatest risk of side effects. Complications of the procedure are similar to those of TURP, and their effects may be more severe. The procedure usually requires a hospital stay of three to five days.

- The da Vinci Prostatectomy (robotic surgery). Thanks to a breakthrough surgical technology, surgeons now widely offer another option for prostatectomy, the da Vinci Prostatectomy. It is interesting that they consider this procedure a minimally invasive treatment. The da Vinci, in my opinion, has been overexaggerated. I still remember some radio and internet marketing slogans pushing this procedure. Pay close attentions to the words "definitive treatments" and "minimally invasive" when reading marketing pitches below.

  "Imagine major surgery performed through the smallest of incisions. Imagine having the benefits of a definitive treatment but with the potential for significantly less pain, a shorter hospital stay, faster return to normal daily activities–as well as the potential for better clinical outcomes".

  "It is important to know that da Vinci surgery does not place a robot to do a surgery on you. Your surgeon is controlling every aspect of the surgery with the assistance of the robot. Only da Vinci overcomes the limitations of both traditional open surgery and conventional minimally invasive surgery. The da Vinci system is a sophisticated robotic platform designed to expand the surgeon's capabilities and, for the first time, offer minimally invasive option to major surgery".

I leave the judgment about the da Vinci system up to you, as it all depends how it has been marketed to you.

With da Vinci, small incisions are used to introduce miniaturized instruments and a high-definition 3-D camera. Seated comfortably at the da Vinci console, your surgeon views a magnified, high-resolution, 3-D image of the surgical site. At the same time, state-of-the-art robotic and computer technologies scale, filter, and seamlessly translate your surgeon's hand movements into precise micro-movements of the da Vinci instruments.

The system cannot be programmed, nor can it make decisions on its own. Rather, the da Vinci system requires that every surgical maneuver be performed with direct input from your surgeon. The robotic prostatectomy system gives surgeons the feeling that their hands are immersed in the patient's body even though they are performing the surgery remotely. All movements of the surgeon's hands are microscaled by the da Vinci robot. As a result, the surgeon feels completely connected to surgery. In the middle of the surgery, I certainly hope that the electricity does not get cut off, and if it does, that the hospital generator is functioning. The da Vinci robotic system provides a much brighter and sharper image than the human eye or any other 3-D laparoscopic prostatectomy endoscope. The system incorporates a proprietary camera that allows the surgeon to easily zoom, rotate, or change the image visualization. The resulting 3-D image is bright and clear, with no flicker as with other laparoscopic systems. Robotic hand simulation and 3-D visualization make the da Vinci robotic system more advanced.

Using the da Vinci system, the surgeon can use "motion scaling," a feature that translates small hand movements outside the patient's body into precise movements inside the body. The surgeon controls the da Vinci robotic prostatectomy robot from the console using natural hand and wrist movements. Proprietary instruments called EndoWrist instruments enable surgeons to reach difficult places in the prostate and suture with precision. Motion scaling is designed to allow greater precision than is normally achievable in open and laparoscopic prostatectomy surgery. Indeed, conventional laparoscopic instruments provide surgeons less flexibility, dexterity, and range of motion. Laparoscopic instruments in use today do not replicate hand movements and cannot perform precise movement and manipulations, such as reaching behind tissues, suturing, and dissection. Added instrument range of motion enhances access and safety while operating in the confined space of the closed chest, abdomen, or pelvis. The system filters out unpredictable movements and tremors inherent in human hands.

In a landmark paper, the largest, most complete study of the return of PSA after radical prostatectomy, Johns Hopkins doctors have developed guidelines to help patients and doctors know what to do if PSA comes back. Their remarkable effort made an elegantly simple chart that accurately predicts a man's risk of developing metastatic cancer. This chart has the potential to revolutionize the way doctors and patients make decisions about what to do next.

"PSA is very sensitive in detecting any recurrence of cancer. That's because only prostate cells make PSA, so if it goes up after a radical prostatectomy, it means prostate cells are still present somewhere. For all intents and purposes, it means that a few cells escaped the prostate before it was removed, and now have grown to the point where they're producing enough PSA to be detected," explains Dr. Walsh of James Brady Urological Institute.

"Fortunately, for most men with organ-confined cancer, this never happens. However, for men who had more advanced disease at the time of surgery, the return of PSA is extremely frightening." Dr. Walsh originated this study to fill what he describes as a "large knowledge gap" for patients and doctors.

The study, published in the *Journal of the American Medical Association*, is based on 10,000 patients with fifteen years of follow-up data between 1982 and 1997. Nearly 2,000 men underwent a radical prostatectorny at Johns Hopkins. Of these, 315 men developed an elevated PSA (defined as being higher than 0.2 nanograms/milliliter). Eleven of these men opted for early hormone therapy and were not included in the study. The remaining 304 men were followed carefully.

On average, it took eight years from the time a man's PSA first went up until he developed metastatic disease, which suggests that there is no need to panic at the first sign of a rise in PSA.

When men see their PSA levels rise again, they think that means the cancer is back and they need to get treated right away. But men often live for years without having the cancer spread. This information will better equip doctors and their patients to decide what treatment, if any, is most appropriate.

This interval between the reappearance of PSA and the first sign of advanced disease can be predicted, the Johns Hopkins researchers found, using three pieces of information:

- The Gleason score of the pathologic specimen (the removed prostate, evaluated by a pathologist after surgery). Is it Gleason 7 or lower or Gleason 8 or greater?
- The time it takes for PSA to come back. Is it less than two years after surgery or more?
- How long does it take for the PSA level to double? Greater or less than ten months?

Using these criteria, men and their doctors can pinpoint the likelihood of developing metastatic disease. For example, if a man has Gleason 7 disease, has his first PSA recurrence more than two years after surgery, and has a PSA doubling time longer than ten months, his likelihood of being free of metastasis at seven years is 82 percent. Conversely, if a man has Gleason 7 disease, but his PSA goes up within two years of surgery, and the time it takes PSA to double is less than ten months, his likelihood of being metastasis-free at seven years is 15 percent.

What if you get PSA anxiety after the surgery?

Let's say that you've had the radical prostatectomy and you happen to read an article on cancer cells coming back after a surgery and you automatically assume that your surgeon did not go far enough. You're terrified that it didn't work. So here you are, a grown man, living in fear of a simple blood test, scared to death that the PSA—an enzyme made only by prostate cells—will come back, but all of your prostate cells are supposed to be gone. Where did they come from?

If you have PSA anxiety, you are not alone. However you should not worry. Sometimes, there is such a thing as too much information.

The only thing that really matters is at what PSA levels does the concentration indicate that the patient has had a recurrence of cancer? The number to take seriously is 0.2 nanograms/milliliter as discussed before. That's something called biochemical recurrence. But even this doesn't mean that a man has symptoms yet. You need to understand that it might take months or even years before there is any clinical physical evidence.

You cannot reliably detect such a small amount as 0.01, and from day to day, the results could vary. It could be 0.03 or maybe even 0.05, and these analytical variations may not mean a thing. It's important that we don't assume anything or take action on a very low level of PSA. In routine practice, because of these analytical variations from day to day, we assume it's the same as nondetectable, or zero.

In 2002, Holmberg, a noted researcher and specialist in the treatment of prostate cancer, presented interim results from a large, randomized trial comparing radical prostatectomy to watchful waiting for the treatment of localized prostate cancer. The trial is virtually without precedent and provides, by far, the best evidence as to the effectiveness of one of the most common surgical operations for cancer.

Interpretation of the trial in the scientific literature appears to have been unequivocal. The journal, *Evidence-Based Medicine*, summarized the results thus: "Radical prostatectomy reduced death from prostate cancer but not all cause mortality. Similarly, a clinical guidelines paper for the U.S. Preventive Services Task Force stated that though surgery reduced 'prostate cancer mortality the groups did not differ in all-cause mortality." The *British Medical Journal* went further, "Watchful waiting as well as surgery for prostate cancer," trumpeted one headline. Another article, entitled, "The operation was a success (but the patients died)," berated the lay press for reporting favorably on surgery. Even the editorial accompanying the original paper, whilst broadly supportive of prostatectomy, stated that there was "no difference between the two groups in overall mortality."

At first glance, the results seem to support the value of prostatectomy. Fifty-three of 347 patients in the prostatectomy group died, and sixteen of them from prostate cancer. From patients in the control group, sixty-two died, including thirty-one deaths from prostate cancer. If around 60,000 prostatectomies are conducted each year in the U.S., and if overall survival is improved by the two to three percent found in this trial, prostatectomy would extend approximately 1,500 American lives each year.

The philosophical basis for never accepting the null hypothesis is the difficulty of proving a negative. We tend to make statements such as, "Extensive searches have failed to find the sea monster," rather than "There is no sea monster" because we cannot rule out the possibility that the monster is hiding somewhere in dark part of the sea that we have yet to look.

In the *British Medical Journal* articles, prostatectomy has also been explained as a surgery that might lower the risk of death from prostate cancer, but increases the risk of death from other causes. This is not uncommon for treatments, such as chemotherapy, that are associated with important toxicities, but would be unusual for a relatively low-risk procedure such as a prostatectomy. Indeed, the cause of death is carefully described in the study report. Although slightly more men in the prostatectomy group died of other causes, a large proportion of the difference is explained by deaths from other cancers.

Approximately 1.5 million men were diagnosed with prostate cancer during a period of three years. If we very conservatively estimate that only 1 percent of those men decided against prostatectomy on the basis of the claim that it has "no effect on overall survival," 15,000 fewer surgeries would have been conducted. Using the updated estimate of a 5 percent decrease in ten-year survival with watchful waiting, 750 men might have died prematurely as the result.

A mistake in the operating room can threaten the life of one patient; a mistake in statistical analysis or interpretation can lead to hundreds of early deaths. So it is perhaps odd that while we allow a doctor to conduct surgery on us only after a few years of training and experience, we give permission to almost anyone to open us up and take out what he or she wants, totally ignoring the statistical data. Moreover, whilst only a surgeon would comment on surgical technique, it seems that anybody, regardless of statistical training, feels confident about commenting on statistical data. If we are to bring the vast efforts of research to fruition and truly practice evidence-based medicine, we must learn to interpret the results of randomized trials appropriately. This will require greater awareness of statistical methods, including the dangers of accepting the null hypothesis and the relative statistical power of overall and cancer-specific survival. Getting these fundamentals right is the very least that we can do for those affected by cancer in the future.

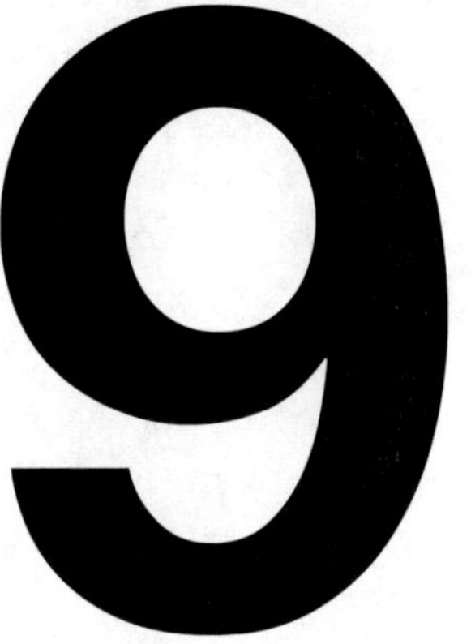

Chapter 9

Genetic Tests and Future Treatments for Prostate Cancer

Could genetic errors play a role in the spread of prostate cancer throughout the body, and is it possible to produce new drug delivery methods with fewer side effects?

Do you have your highlighter ready? Let's start.

Even though a few companies in U.S. already offer genetic testing, it is still a very new concept in this country and scientists agree that more research is necessary as the test includes only five out of all the genes that may affect prostate cancer risk.

In Britain, where every year more than 32,000 men are diagnosed and 10,000 die from the disease, a genetic test that identifies men most at risk of prostate cancer is already available. British doctors use PROGENSA

PCA3, the world's first gene-based urine test, to spot the disease in its earliest stages, before it has become dangerously advanced or has spread throughout the body. This test measures a genetic chemical, messenger RNA, which transfers DNA "instructions" from the PCA3 gene. Elevated scores indicate prostate cancer presence.

New clinical data from study of 570 men published in the *Journal of Urology* supports the PROGENSA PCA3 as a valid prostate cancer diagnostic tool, which provides valuable information helping with correct diagnosis.

Scientists began work on the test following a landmark study of nearly 2,000 cancer patients, which found seven previously unknown genetic markers that are linked to the disease. Each one raises the risk of prostate cancer by around 60 percent.

The findings, reported in the journal, *Nature Genetics*, paved the way for the first reliable screening test for men at high risk of the disease, and might also lead to new drug therapies for the condition.

The latest work, funded by Cancer Research UK, identified genetic markers that may be carried by more than half of all men with prostate cancer.

The markers were discovered by comparing the DNA of men with prostate cancer with DNA from healthy patients. They collected DNA samples from 1,854 men who had been diagnosed with prostate cancer by the age of sixty or younger or who had a family history of the disease. They then gathered DNA from 1,894 men with similar lifestyles who were known to have a low risk of prostate cancer from PSA tests.

By comparing the DNA from the two groups, the scientists identified seven "spelling mistakes" in the genetic code that were strongly linked to the cancer. One gene, called MSMB, seems to play a role in prostate cancer returning after treatment but could also be used to screen for the disease. A second gene, called LMTK2, is a promising target for new drugs to treat the disease.

The next challenge is to predict who will develop the disease. If it works, doctors will be able to single out men who are most at risk for closer monitoring at a much earlier stage. Just imagine that your son, on his twentieth birthday, receives a call from his urologist that tells him that he falls under the Gleason 8 category ten years from now.

Laurie Whelan, a sixty-nine-year-old father of three from London, took part in the study after doctors discovered he had advanced prostate cancer. He was persuaded to take the test by his younger brother, who already had prostate cancer. Their older brother had previously died of the disease. "It turned out that I had a locally advanced cancer which had reached the outside of the gland," he said.

His cancer was too far developed for surgery to help, but instead, he received hormone treatment and radiotherapy. These areas are currently being researched at the Prince of Wales Hospital's Oncology Research Center with the funding from the U.S. Army Medical Research and Materiel Command which has a mandate to 'provide solutions to medical problems' for military personnel.

The first study will investigate the role of genes thought to be involved in the spread of prostate cancer to other, more life-threatening parts of the body, while the second project is concerned with new treatments for prostate cancer that seek to target cancer cells while ignoring their healthy neighbors.

Researchers already know that errors in genetic material, or DNA, are responsible for all cancers. Previous studies showed that additional genetic errors might also explain why some prostate cancers metastasize, or spread throughout the body, while the vast majority of prostate cancers that lack these errors remain slow growing and are less likely to cause harm.

One of the main suspects involved in the spread of prostate cancer is a gene called p53. It's thought that genetic mistakes or mutations within certain regions of the p53 gene might make the cancer more likely to spread to the bone, the most common site of metastasis in advanced prostate cancer patients. Using human prostate cancer cells grown in the laboratory, the research involves creating a series of artificial prostate cancers, each carrying a different error within the p53 gene.

That enables the researchers to determine whether the genetic mutation of the p53 gene allows the cancer cell to spread and grow inside the patient's bone or not.

The second project will examine if there are ways to make chemotherapy more effective and to protect patients from some of the debilitating side effects of the cancer drugs.

Let's get a bit deeper into the subject of gene p53 (area 53!).

Gene p53 keeps watch over DNA during cell division, and it is called "the tumor suppressor gene p53," which in its natural state is known as "wild type p53." "Wild type p53" could actually be the name of a nightclub, where all the crazy cancer cells go dancing, but for now, let's keep the nightclub closed, as the wild type p53 may block tumor growth by inducing apoptosis (programmed cell death) and by causing reversible arrest in the cell cycle.

P53-dependent apoptosis seems to be the mechanism for the antitumor effect of radiation and certain chemotherapy drugs.

Mutations in p53 are detected in more than 50 percent of all human cancers such as lung, breast, brain, and bladder. Cancer cells with mutated p53 are more resistant to chemotherapy and radiation therapy and provide a genetic basis for drug resistance. We also know that cancers with frequent mutations in p53 respond poorly to therapy, whereas cancers that rarely have p53 mutations respond well to therapy.

We now are entering the age of genetic therapy to treat cancer. The rationale for this is that cancers are DNA disorders. Defects in our DNA either turn cell division on or do not turn off cell division. Genes responsible for turning on cell division in a cancer cell are termed oncogenes. Genes that function to turn off aberrant cell growth are called tumor suppressor genes. Defects in these genes create and perpetuate cancers. New approaches to cancer utilizing genetic therapy involve manipulating these genes to halt cancer. Studies to date indicate that a cell must sustain damage to one oncogene and three tumor suppressor genes to create malignancy.

Telomeres are short strips of DNA that are found at the tips of chromosomes. A young cell has more than a 1,000 telomeres. During cell division, the cell loses ten to twenty telomeres. With continued cell division, the telomere number drops to a certain level and cell division stops. The cell has aged, and cell death occurs. This is, in essence, a built-in biological clock that affects all normal cells in our body.

There is an enzyme called telomerase that protects the telomere chain, thus prolonging the life of cell. Telomerase is found only in two cell types: sperm cells and cancer cells. Telomerase, in essence, immortalizes these cell types. We should be working on drugs that inhibit telomerase production or block its action to destroy the cancer cell.

Angiogenesis relates to the formation of new blood vessels. Cancer growth is restricted to less than one million cells in the absence of new blood vessels. Tumor growth is therefore angiogenesis dependent. This has been histologically confirmed in studies on prostate cancer correlating the number of vessels seen with the microscope with the rate of metastasis.

The cancer cell has the ability to trigger blood vessel formation, which feeds the tumor and allows for its spread. However, a protein called Thrombospondin (TS) has been discovered to inhibit blood vessel growth. TS appear to be regulated by the p53 oncogene. Mutations in p53 may turn off TS, resulting in angiogenesis and further tumor growth.

Nm23, a nonmetastasis gene, helps mature cells stop dividing and allows the cells to arrange themselves in an orderly fashion. Nm23 given to mice with tumors resulted in a reduction in formation of metastasis by 90 percent. MTS1 is a multiple tumor suppressor gene. Defects in MTS1 may cause various cancers such as lung, breast, melanoma, and brain tumors. Treatment with MTS1 may inhibit tumor growth.

The idea here is that if we cannot kill those rascals, we should teach them to be nice, and friendly. Research is needed in designing drugs that convert mutant p53 to normal (wild type) p53. We need to learn how to genetically splice wild type p53 into p53 negative tumors. We can learn to destroy the cancer cell with drugs that block telomerase action or inhibit its production. Other areas of pursuit involve inhibition of angiogenesis with synthetic Thrombospondin or stopping tumor growth with MTS1.

P53, a tumor suppressor gene, helps regulate the cell cycle. It plays a key role in ensuring that damaged cells are destroyed by apoptosis (programmed cell death). P53 is the most commonly mutated gene associated with cancer.

Normally, if anything damages the DNA (genetic code) in the body's cells, protein p53 puts a brake on the cell cycle. Cellular repair systems set to work and, if necessary, get rid of the damaged cells by apoptosis (a form of cell suicide).

P53's job is cell cycle arrest. But if p53 itself has mutated and no longer works properly, proliferation of damaged cells goes unchecked. Cancer and spread of cancer can occur.

Chemotherapy, as it is being used by doctors loosely due to misconception of killing only the cancer cells, must cease to exist in our hospitals. It was developed more than fifty years ago, and the doctors have been limited by the amount of drugs they can give a patient because of the toxic effect on other cells. In the future, there should be ways to target chemotherapy directly to the prostate and leave healthy cells in other organs unscathed, as it is the case today.

In this case, a cancer drug that requires chemical conversion must be created and tested. This pro-drug has to have no side effects and should kill cancer cells. The trick has been to create a genetic switch that only works inside prostate cells to reactivate the pro-drug into its lethal form to assassinate the cancer cells.

The three-year study at the Oncology Research Center involves inserting this artificial gene into a patient's prostate cancer cells, using a friendly virus to carry the genetic cargo as an insider spy. So far, the results have been impressive, with growth rates significantly reduced in prostate cancers grown in the laboratory.

Chapter 10

Conclusion

Our human body is made by our creator, and walking by faith and not by sight is the key when you hear that you have prostate cancer confirmed on the third opinion.

It is time to complete this book, which I hope has given you a big push to do more research and obtain at least three opinions before allowing your surgeon open you up, just to find out later that it was a mistake.

As history has shown, doctors can be wrong. Well-accepted health truths can be wrong. And ideas that have seemed completely crazy have later on turned out to be true.

So how can you know who to believe and whose professional opinion you can trust? You can't.

To finalize this book I am including the most important aspect: faith.

When I interviewed patients in different stages of prostate cancer I noticed that they all have one thing in common: worry. Not so much about themselves, but about their loved ones. "What will happen to my kids, my wife if I die", "Why me?" or "Where is God?" often came to their minds. Little did they know that God is omnipresent. Our mind is too limited to comprehend it, but God does provide the way to overcome the difficulties we encounter in our lives.

I tried to mix the subjects of this book with humor in order to remove the tension and worry. At no time did I think the serious subjects discussed here were funny.

"It is beyond our comprehension," I said as I laid hands on the forehead of a cancer patient that was given only a few weeks to live since the chemotherapy was no longer the solution. I cried as I was praying and asking God to intervene. After I went home, I could not sleep the whole night, thinking that we humans try to understand and use the "why" word quite often, but we seem to forget that not everything in this universe is comprehendible. Why 90 percent of the terrorist acts around the world originate in Muslim countries? Why do so many tsunamis and earthquakes happen in Indonesia? Why do the drought and famine afflict the poorest countries in Africa? Why AIDS plagues primarily people of African countries? The fact is that no one on this planet can explain it.

For decades, the scientists have been trying to prove that our existence within the galaxy is nothing but a coincidence and the presence of God is just an illusion and fairytales that have been made up in the past. How is all this relevant to the subject of this book, you may ask? Well, if we believe that there is a Creator that made us, then we, regardless of religion, can be in full communication with that Creator via communications (prayers), and that Creator can be in full control of our destiny. Our requests could be in our prayers, and the responses for those prayers are forthcoming. If there is no Creator to communicate with and the reason for our existence is according to the Big Bang theory, then all our prayers will absolutely have no results.

Interestingly, there were a few experiments by scientists that provide evidence for the power of prayer. Those experiments involving human DNA have proved that our DNA can and does directly affect our physical world. This is what the Law of Attraction proponents have been saying for more than a century.

There is an enormous amount of evidence to support the existence of energy fields in the rapidly growing field of energy psychology.

One group of experiments was actually done by the military. They collected leukocytes (white blood cells) from donors and placed them into chambers so that their electrical charges could be measured. Then the donor was placed in a different room in the same building as the chamber containing his DNA. He was then subjected to emotional stimulation, using video clips.

Both the donor and his DNA were monitored for their electrical responses.

As the donor exhibited emotional peaks or valleys, the DNA exhibited electrical responses at the same time. There was no lag time—no transition time. The matches were exact and instantaneous.

The experiment was repeated at longer distances between donor and DNA, up to 50 miles. In every case, the donor and his DNA showed the same effect, simultaneously.

What can this mean?

Gregg Braden, a scientist, visionary and scholar internationally renowned as a pioneer in bridging science and spirituality, has the following interpretation:

"Living cells communicate through a previously unrecognized form of energy that is not affected by time or distance. This is a non-local form of energy that already exists everywhere, all the time."

Another experiment was done by the Institute of Heartmath, a recognized, global leader in emotional physiology, stress management and the physiology of heart-brain research, and it involved human placental DNA, which is the most pristine form of DNA. It was again placed into a container from which they could measure its changes.

Twenty-eight vials of DNA were given to 28 researchers, who were specially trained in how to generate and feel strong emotions on demand. The results were astounding.

Each DNA sample changed shape according to its researcher's feelings:

- When the researchers felt love, joy, and gratitude, the DNA responded by relaxing: the strands unwound and actually lengthened.
- When the researchers felt anger, fear, frustration, or stress, the DNA tightened up, became shorter and even switched off many of its codes!
- When the researchers felt love, joy, and gratitude again, the codes switched back on.

What could it mean for your health? Think about it.

If your DNA can affect all of the energy around you, what could you potentially create in your life if you focus on the things you truly want?

The possibilities have no limits …

- No matter what viruses or bacteria are floating around you, you can stay well by staying in positive feelings such as of love, joy and gratitude.
- You can stay safe and grounded, regardless of your external situation.
- You have the ultimate power to create the health you want.
- You can reverse the cancer cell threatening division and get cured by your positive attitude and rock-solid belief that your immune system working perfectly fine to wipe out the bad guys.

The key is to stay in the right emotional state, which could be achieved by faith and deep prayers. If you are having a trouble to get into that positive emotional state you need to try and connect with God.

We will always need water, oxygen, and food for preserving our flesh, but what about our emotional being, our psychic, our soul? Just as our body needs nutrients to survive and thrive, our soul needs the nutrients (communication and prayers with our creator) as well.

There is such a thing as a soul, spirit, energy, or whatever you call it, inside of you; and whatever it is, it must be fed or it gradually dies. Our prayers and communications with our Creator will keep our soul alive. If you were to win a lottery today and you wanted to buy a car, what would you buy? Well, since the majority of the people that are reading this book are men, I assume it will be a Ferrari, Rolls Royce or Mercedes, right?

Now, let's say that you found your new Ferrari at an 80 percent discount, it was delivered to your home, you were given the key and it sits on your driveway until you find out that it does not have an engine. How would you feel? "Wait a minute, this is a scam," you say to the salesperson.

"But, sir, why do you think that we are selling you the car at 20 percent of the actual price?" the salesperson responds.

"Because I thought I got a good deal," you say.

"No, sir I can refund you the money if you return the car," the salesperson says.

"Okay, I will bring it back, but just out of curiosity, what made you think that I would want to buy a car without the engine?" you ask.

"Because, sir, some of our customers want to show off to their friends by just keeping the car on the driveway," he says.

You say to yourself, "Hey, this is not a bad idea."

The Ferrari, just like any other car, needs the engine to move from your driveway. The same engine that is called our soul or spirit also is within us; otherwise our flesh will not survive. What you use for making the exterior of the Ferrari shiny and beautiful, such as paint and wax, is not the same as oil and water that its engine needs. Similarly with humans–the type of food we need for our body is different from the food we need for our soul. Our spiritual food is the prayer.

A lot of people that you and I know have live body, but their soul is either dead or borderline. Have you heard of "speaking in tongues"? It is a form of communication between our soul and God. It is described in the Bible, and you can find such practices in charismatic churches where one can speak in tongues, and another can interpret it. It is a language that partly similar to African and Latin, and the person that prays does not understand the words, as such words basically connect the soul to the Creator. Once that communication line is open between you and your Creator, be ready for miracles as the impossible become possible.

If the soul is borderline dead, the devil can then take over, and I am sure you have heard of devil-possessed individuals. It is mind-boggling, but I have seen those people in Guatemala during an evangelist visit and have observed driving out the demons, just like the exorcism.

What is the point in all this? With God everything is possible, especially curing your prostate cancer. Your soul, once in line with the will of God, can generate p53's genes and completely reverse the cancer cells to good cells.

There are many things in this life that can affect our predisposition to prostate cancer.

Defective genes may be inherited from parents as occurs in early onset colorectal cancer, and cancers of the prostate, breast, lung, and brain. Acquired genetic defects may be induced as a result of viral infection as seen with HIV, hepatitis C, B, and E-B viruses, to name a few.

Environmental toxins, such as insecticides, cigarette smoke, asbestos, benzene, aflatoxin, radon, and vinyl chloride, have well-known associations with various types of cancers. Combinations of exposures to cigarette smoke and asbestos, for example, further increase the risk of cancer. These toxic exposures therefore are synergistic in their carcinogenesis.

Various electromagnetic energies may induce genetic damage. Radiation from sun exposure, nuclear fallout, and excessive X-ray exposure are known factors that increase risk of cancer.

Apoptosis-regulating genes are believed to play an important role in the development and progression of prostate cancer. They are viewed as a potential target for future treatment strategies.

Knowledge is power, and this power along with the power of prayer will get you through any trials.

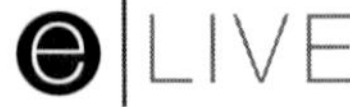

listen|imagine|view|experience

AUDIO BOOK DOWNLOAD INCLUDED WITH THIS BOOK!

In your hands you hold a complete digital entertainment package. In addition to the paper version, you receive a free download of the audio version of this book. Simply use the code listed below when visiting our website. Once downloaded to your computer, you can listen to the book through your computer s speakers, burn it to an audio CD or save the file to your portable music device (such as Apple s popular iPod) and listen on the go!

How to get your free audio book digital download:

1. Visit www.tatepublishing.com and click on the e|LIVE logo on the home page.
2. Enter the following coupon code: 81b2-9ab6-31aa-e794-e9a6-41ab-d310-ead3
3. Download the audio book from your e|LIVE digital locker and begin enjoying your new digital entertainment package today!

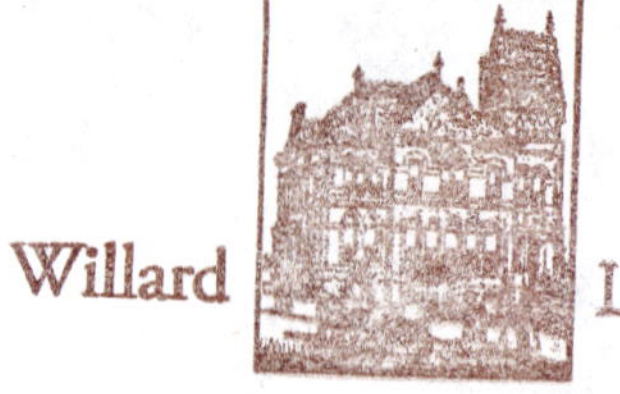